T0078097

An Analysis of Independent Restaurants Featuring Organic Food in Metropolitan Cities in the United States

A Quantitative Approach

Nina Moore; Tarnue Johnson

authorHOUSE®

AuthorHouse™
1663 Liberty Drive
Bloomington, IN 47403
www.authorhouse.com
Phone: 1 (800) 839-8640

Published by AuthorHouse 02/07/2017

ISBN: 978-1-5246-6005-5 (sc)
ISBN: 978-1-5246-6006-2 (e)

Print information available on the last page.

Any people depicted in stock imagery provided by Thinkstock are models, and such images are being used for illustrative purposes only. Certain stock imagery © Thinkstock.

This book is printed on acid-free paper.

Contents

Dedication

This book is dedicated to all those who have now become convinced in the face of mounting evidence that the embrace of organic foods is a reasoned path to pursue in the 21st century, in an age of the application of ever intensive methods of food production and mass consumption. Above all, the book is dedicated to the people of Belize and Liberia as they seek to thrive and prosper in their national strivings.

Acknowledgements

We would like to extent our deepest gratitude and sincere appreciation to those who reviewed the manuscript and provided useful feedback. These included Dr. Robert Castaneda, Dr. Harold O'Kere, Dr. James Carter and Dr. Sherry Haynes. Thus, it goes without saying that the feedback and critical comments provided by these scholars only helped to enrich the texture of our conclusions, scope, analytical rigor and breadth of our analyses and critical concerns reported in this book.

A Tribute to One of the Authors

From the humblest beginnings, to scholar, Nina M. Moore has traversed the explosive and dynamic landscape of her surroundings. Men and women are often defined by what they are able to accomplish. There has not been a more critical time in our society for police officers. In the midst of police work, with its constant upheaval and controversy, a phoenix has arisen to help put forth a scholarly effort, which will last for generations. Kudos to a strong, positive woman who has outperformed the expectations placed upon her. May her example shine as a beacon of hope for young women everywhere.

Dr. James Darious Carter

About the Authors

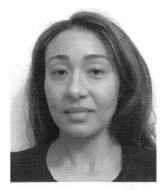

Dr. Nina M. Moore obtained her BA degree in business administration from DeVry University in Chicago, IL (2000-03). Dr. Moore upon completing her undergraduate degree entered a career in law enforcement, where she currently serves in the Chicago area (2003-current). While serving as law enforcement officer, she continued her education at St. Xavier University in Chicago, IL, where shed obtained an MA in Business Administration (2007-08). Dr. Moore completed her Doctorate in Business Administration (DBA) at Argosy University in Chicago, IL (2009-16). Dr. Moore has also served as project manager, which involved leading a team of community stakeholders in the context of community policing and public safety in Chicago.

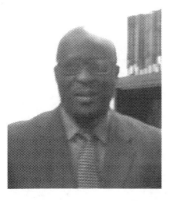

Dr. Tarnue Johnson obtained an MA in Political Economy from Middlesex Universityin London, UK (1992-94). Dr. Johnson completed a Postgraduate Certificate in Adult Education at the Institute of Education, University College London (1995-96). He spent a year doing postgraduate studies in Educational Research, Policy and Planning at the University of Manchester in Manchester, UK (1997-98).

Dr. Johnson completed his Doctorate in Business Administration (DBA) at Argosy University with concentration in management (2007-11). He also completed Postdoctoral Studies in Public Policy at Northwestern University (2015). Dr. Johnson has authored and co-authored eleven books including the current publication with leading American and African scholars and intellectuals. He has also written and published several peer-reviewed articles in reputable journals. Dr. Johnson has served as Senior Lecturer in business and economics at Kendall College in Chicago, Doctoral Advisor at Argosy University and Associate Vice President for Academic Support Services at Tubman University in Liberia. He was recently appointed as Head of the Graduate School of Professional Studies at Cuttington University in Liberia.

A Poem on Organic Food

Man Revises our Creator's Design
By
Dann Ann Smith-Johnson

(**Source**: http://www.poetrysoup.com/poem/manrevisesourcreatorsdesign 86178)

Improve quality of food shall surely benefit man
Quantity increases will feed the hungry and poor
To the common man, at first, it sounds like the perfect plan.
Gene changed gorgeous fruits adorn the produce store.

Genetically change super plants manipulate God's world.
Seeming positive at first, scheming power at its worst—
Undermine the little man; devious research unfurled.
Appearing beneficial, redesign is by greed cursed.

Third world countries co-align as those in power hold their hands.
Their research advancements are supported from sea to seas.
Genetic exploration changes God designed croplands.
New producers thwart small farmers; they manipulate bees.

Homestead farmers feel the pain; sterile seeds do not grow plants.
Meanwhile the power hungry cannot quench greed's growing thirst.
Generational practices work hard to keep their stance.
But into microscopic life new laws of order soon burst.

Nina Moore; Tarnue Johnson

Lobbyists seek to stop homesteaders that grow their own crops.
Sterile seeds and dying bees are the super's starting spot.
Rooftop beehives and small farm home-crops try to mend teardrops.
Changing God's world is the backdrop to a shifting hilltop.

Preface

Official Government Statistics and recent research reports in various Journals of Consumer Studies indicate that the preference for organic food is becoming ubiquitous as consumers who can afford seek to shift away from processed foods and others they perceive as harmful to their health. It is doubtless to note that the dramatic transformation in the pattern of demand in this market segment has been occasioned thanks to the growing health challenges that consumers faced.

However, in the face of this growing demand, there is also a paucity of data on the organic food business. Hence, because of the problem of limited information, it is difficult to accurately discern and investigate the interplay of variables that affect the current pattern of demand for organic foods, let alone how independent restaurants are positioning themselves to furnish the burgeoning demand in this market.

The authors hope that the current book is a timely response to some of these challenges. Readers should note that in writing this book, our working assumption hinged upon the notion that public policy makers should seek to expand the demand and supply of organic foods to benefit all segments of society, especially those who live in what some called "food deserts" across metropolitan centers in the United States. Our collaborative reflection, nuanced and critical examination of data led us to embrace the scientific assumption that the consumption of healthy foods is one of the positive ingredients that undergird the formation of a wholesome functioning society.

These imperatives are among the several that shaped the epistemological and methodological foundations of our belief that a study of this nature to fill in some of these gaps in scholarly and popular knowledge, information, and understanding could not be more relevant at this historical point in time. The various chapters of this book dwelled essentially on the ethical, managerial and microeconomic factors (average costs, revenue, risk-taking, profit etc.) that affect leadership and organizational success in the context of niched independent restaurants in the hospitality industry across metropolitan areas in the United States.

Several chapters, for example, stressed the fact that additional empirical studies may also be needed---despite current efforts----to address some of the questions associated with the factors that affect the successes and failures of independent organic restaurants to breach the gap in scholarship. We suggested that the aim of such studies could be to consider a host of other independent variables that we did not include in a study very limited in scope as ours.

As mentioned earlier, the results of our study reported in this book also analyzed factors that influence independent restaurants featuring organic food in metropolitan cities in the United States. Those factors examined included profits, average costs, menu category, and the number of customers served per week at each of the independent organic restaurants in the sample. Data on profits and average costs covered only a one-year period. The study adopted a survey research approach and used a purposive sample of (N = 36) participants.

The targeted population for the study was independent restaurants that had been in operation for over five years and offered organic food on their menus. Data analyses were performed using Pearson correlation, regression, and one-way ANOVA. The study reports and discusses the implications of the research findings for professional practice, organizational leadership, and restaurant success. We strongly hope that this book will be useful as an important academic resource to management scholars, students and practitioners in the food and hostility industries. We also truly hope that readers will thoroughly enjoy reading this book despite its technical nature and analytical orientation.

Organization of the Book

This book is the result of an adaptation of original research conducted by Nina M. Moore in partial fulfillment of a Doctorate Degree in Business Administration from Argosy University. Results of research reported in the book invariably focused on the factors that influence the relative success and failure of independent restaurants in some metropolitan cities in the United States. The book is divided into five chapters. Chapter One sought to provide the problem background of this study in terms of the underlying reasons that led to the selection of this topic. The underlying research questions that undergirded this study were also included in chapter one.

Similarly, the chapter provided the purpose and nature of this study. The statement of the problem was also provided. Next, the chapter presented the significance of the study and the research hypotheses. The delimitations and limitations of the study were provided as well as the definitions of terms.

Chapter Two sought to explore the research literature that forms the theoretical basis for the research. The literature review chapter discussed prior empirical and theoretical studies that have focused on independent restaurants. The literature review examines two broad conceptual and theoretical perspectives that were used as a basis for the study. The first focuses on the factors that determine the success and failure of independent restaurants. The second focuses on the influence of leadership factors on the organizational climate of independent restaurants, including those that feature organic food.

This chapter also attempts to identify gaps in prior academic studies. This researcher suggests that to a large extent, it was critical awareness of these gaps that informed the rationale for this study. The final section of this chapter focuses on the summary and conclusion.

Chapter Three presented the methodological framework that undergirded this study. It also presented a restatement of the research problem. The chapter further discussed the research design, including the characteristics and type of survey instrument adopted. The methodological assumptions that ensured validity of the research findings were also established. The chapter presented the selection of the research participants as well as data analysis. Furthermore, the chapter discussed the validity and reliability of the study.

In addition, the ethical considerations that were the guideposts for this study were discussed in this chapter. Chapter Four provided the results of the data analysis in an attempt to explain some of the factors that affect independent restaurants that feature organic foods in the United States. Descriptive statistics as well as inferential statistics are provided and analyzed in this chapter.

The chapter also discussed the results of the data analysis in an attempt to explain some of the factors that affect independent restaurants that feature organic foods in the United States. Chapter Five discussed the research findings in the context of existing empirical studies. The chapter also presented some of the factors that account for both the relative success and failure of restaurants in the niched independent sectors.

Further, the discussion in this chapter urged scholars to go beyond the construct of rate of return to focus on other quantitative and qualitative factors that account for success in independent restaurants. This chapter put forth the notion that studies about the factors that undergird the successes or failures of independent restaurants should include quantitative and qualitative variables that transcend financial modeling. The chapter presented the results of hypotheses testing, which was performed using correlation and regression analyses.

Chapter One
Introduction

Introduction

This chapter will provide the problem background of this study in terms of the underlying reasons that led to the selection of this topic. The underlying research questions for this study will also be introduced. Similarly, the chapter will provide the purpose and nature of this study. The statement of the problem will also be provided. Next, the chapter will present the significance of the study and the research hypotheses. The delimitations and limitations of the study will be provided as well as the definitions of terms.

Problem Background

This study was conducted in the tradition established by researchers that have focused on the factors that influence the success and failure of independent restaurants (Agarwal & Dahm, 2015; Camillo, Connolly, & Kim, 2008; Kareklas, Carlson, & Muehling, 2014; Parsa, Self, Njite, & King, 2005; Parsa, van der Rest, Smith, Parsa, & Bujisic, 2015). Thus, this study analyzed the perspective of owners/operators and factors that influence independent restaurants featuring organic food in metropolitan cities in the United States.

One of the driving inspirations for this study was the fact that it is becoming harder for many consumers to identify the right foods to eat (Organic Trade Association, 2016). This view has been reechoed essentially by consumers, The Food and Drug Administration (FDA), and scholars focusing on trends in the food and hospitality industries (Boger, 1995; Economic Information Bulletin, 2009; FDA, 2016; Gregory et al., 2014).

Readers, public policy experts, management scholars, and students might also want to ask the essential question: "Why is this particular phenomenon a problem?" The authors suggest that this is a problem because of the potential public health challenges associated with consumers not knowing the difference between the health benefits of certain categories of foods and others that might pose untold risks. We currently live in a changing world when it comes to the processes and labeling affecting the food industry. Hence, given the fact that the food landscape has changed, consumers are now clamoring for organic food because of its perceived beneficial health effects (The European Food Information Council, 2013). This has made the preference for organic foods a major factor affecting the growth of independent restaurants that focus on organic foods.

It has been reported that organic foods have become increasingly prominent among consumers in terms of the shelf space they occupy in the produce, dairy, and specialty aisles of most mainstream food retailers in the United States (*Economic Information Bulletin*, 2009). The *Economic Information Bulletin* (2009) also reported that the marketing boom of organic foods increased their retail sales to $21 billion in 2008 from $3.6 billion in 1997.

Many independent restaurants in various categories have taken advantage of this new pattern of opportunities in the food marketplace by positioning themselves to provide services that cater to customers in this market segment. We identified at least one example of the many documentaries that have appeared in recent years attempting to promote ideas around concepts such as the necessity for environmental stewardship and healthy living through educating consumers about the value of nutrients consumed from whole foods and plants versus animal products (*Forks Over Knives*, 2011).

The Food and Drug Administration (FDA) is a federal agency responsible for overseeing and regulating food and drugs for most of the U.S. food supply. The FDA is responsible for protecting public health by ensuring the safety and security of our nation's food supply (Boger, 1995; FDA, 2016; *Economic Information Bulletin*, 2009; Rahkovsky & Anekwe, 2014).

The United States Department of Agriculture (USDA) protects and promotes healthier food consumption through educating the public, food testing, implementing recalls and safety alerts, and applying stringent rules and regulations to the inspection of domestic and imported produces (USDA, 2016).

As with many products on the market, several factors affect consumers' purchase decisions. For example, Kareklas et al. (2014), Aertsens et al. (2011), and Kriwy et al. (2012) suggested that attitudes, beliefs, and behaviors are factors that influence organic food purchase decisions. We would suggest that people who consume organic food tend to be concerned about their personal health as well as the welfare of animals and the environment.

Another food organization, the Organic Trade Association (OTA; 2016), indicated that organic foods have gained a steady growth in popularity within the last 10 years and currently are the fastest growing food sector in the United States. Yet organic food ingredients within restaurants are still very limited and hard to locate. However, this problem has been somewhat modified. For example, Improvonia—an application (app) that allows suppliers to order specific organic food—has also done much to increase awareness about organic food (OTA, 2016).

The sales of Whole Foods—a pioneer of the organic food industry in terms of selling organic food to consumers in grocery stores—are on a decline due to increased competition from other grocery stores, such as Wal-Mart and Kroger (Bloomberg (2015) & Patton (2015). The "Wal-Mart effect" has assisted in lending positive beliefs and attitudes to the concepts of cooking and consuming organic food. This fact only demonstrates the growing demand for organic food purchase, not just in supermarkets, although challenges still remain (Wells, 2013), but in independent restaurants as well.

However, one should note that this growing demand is being met and that there are several factors that impinge upon restaurants that sell organic food to meet this burgeoning demand. Thus, the central problem that this study analyzed was how these factors have affected independent restaurants in carrying out their business operations (Dimitri & Green, 2002). To achieve this analytical task, the study examined the interaction of the dependent and independent variables using correlation and regression analysis. One-way ANOVA was also used to determine the differences between mean responses among the three groups of restaurants regarding their average cost per item on the menu. Readers should note that some of the central variables in question have been defined below in the section on definitions of terms.

Purpose and Nature of the Study

The purpose of this study was to investigate the phenomenon of organic foods sold in independent restaurants. Past and present studies have suggested that independent restaurants have a higher rate of failure during their first five years in operation (Angelo, 2008; Parsa et al., 2011). For small restaurants and niche restaurants, this realization can be even more challenging. Present studies have suggested that business owners play the most important role in the success or failure of a business, even when featuring organic food (Carvalho & Silva, 2014; Connolly & Kim, 2008).

This research was conducted within the framework of a quantitative study and with independent restaurant owners who have been in operation for over five years and serve organic food. A survey and purposive sample allowed the researcher to collect quantitative data on owners' demographics, average costs and profits associated with their business operations, leadership traits, and classification of their independent restaurants into Quick Service, Midservice, and Upscale. Other variables investigated included participants' thoughts on organic food, mode of advertisement of their restaurants, number of days their restaurants were opened per week, seating capacity, life cycle of their restaurants, financial investments, and emotional attachment by restaurant owners and managers to their businesses.

Statement of the Problem

One of the problems and challenges that invariably provided the rationale for this research is the current paucity of data on the organic food businesses. Some scholars have posited that food is being purchased on a relatively large scale (see Budhwar, 2004). However, this author also observed that there exists limited survey research that investigates the pattern of demand in this sector (Budhwar, 2004; Jinghan, 2007). Compared to the recent past, consumers today are taking more care to know where their food comes from and what is in that food. The problem is that little research has been conducted to investigate the variables affecting the current pattern of demand for organic food, let alone how independent restaurants are positioning themselves to furnish the need in this market (Budhwar, 2004).

Budhwar (2004) indicated that gathering data on organic food is an uphill task. One should recognize the fact that those consumers who are health and nutrition conscious possess necessary awareness and knowledge of food and labels. However, for those consumers who are not health conscious, labels may not have an effect when selecting a lower calorie item from the menu (Ellison, 2013). Because of these and other reasons, a study of organic food will fill in some of these gaps in scholarly and popular knowledge, as further information and understanding could not be more relevant at this point in time. Empirical research studies may also be needed to address some of the questions associated with the factors that affect the successes and failures of independent organic restaurants, as there is a paucity of empirical and theoretical studies in this field.

Significance of the Study

This study which investigates the phenomenon of organic foods sold in independent restaurants will contribute to the research literature on the perceptions of independent restaurant owners and managers that provide organic food on their menus. The study specifically sought to focus on an analysis of profits and how they influence independent restaurants that feature organic food, as well as how those factors influence their classification into the three types referred to in this study. In addition, this study focused on the sources of success and failure of independent restaurants and how leadership traits (see Appendix 3) affect other variables, such as average cost, employee training, and honesty.

We also note that the study's findings will provide important insight for those entrepreneurs already in the food restaurant industry who want to become more specialized in using organic food products. We anticipate this study will provide an invaluable resource for those students who already have a sense of management and are interested in the dynamics of the organic food restaurant factors.

Research Questions

The following research questions guided the research process:

1. To what extent do factors such as the average cost associated with the sale of each meal, profits, and life cycle influence independent restaurants that feature organic food in metropolitan cities in the United States?
2. To what extent do average cost associated with the sale of each meal and profits influence the classification of independent restaurants that feature organic food in metropolitan cities in the United States into Quick Service, Midservice, and Upscale?

Statement of Research Hypotheses

Four research hypotheses were developed to guide this study. The research hypotheses have been duly correlated with their corresponding research questions in the text below. The central objective of these hypotheses was to help investigate the factors that affect independent restaurants that feature organic food. These research hypotheses are as follows:

H_{1o}: The average cost associated with the sale of each meal has no impact on the classification of independent restaurants featuring organic food.

H_{1a}: The average cost associated with the sale of each meal has an impact on the classification of independent restaurants featuring organic food.

H_{2o}: The average cost associated with the sale of each meal has no impact on the days of operation of independent restaurants featuring organic food.

H_{2a}: The average cost associated with the sale of each meal has a significant impact on the days of operation of independent restaurants featuring organic food.

H_{3o}: The profits from the operations of independent restaurants featuring organic food have no relationship with their classification.

H_{3a}: The profits from the operations of independent restaurants featuring organic food have a significant relationship with their classification.

H_{4o}: The life cycle of independent restaurants featuring organic food has no impact on their profits.

H_{4a}: The life cycle of independent restaurants featuring organic food has a significant impact on their profits.

Statement of the Research Questions with Their Corresponding Research Hypotheses

RQ1: To what extent do factors such as the average cost associated with the sale of each meal and life cycle influence independent restaurants that feature organic food in metropolitan cities in the United States?

H_{2o}: The average cost associated with the sale of each meal has no impact on the days of operation of independent restaurants featuring organic food. (RQ1)

H_{2a}: The average cost associated with the sale of each meal has a significant impact on the days of operation of independent restaurants featuring organic food. (RQ1)

H_{4o}: The life cycle of independent restaurants featuring organic food has no impact on their profits. (RQ1)

H_{4a}: The life cycle of independent restaurants featuring organic food has a significant impact on their profits. (RQ1)

RQ2: To what extent do average cost associated with the sale of each meal and profits influence the classification of independent restaurants that feature organic food in metropolitan cities in the United States into Quick Service, Midservice, and Upscale?

H_{1o}: The average cost associated with the sale of each meal has no impact on the classification of independent restaurants featuring organic food. (RQ2)

H_{1a}: The average cost associated with the sale of each meal has an impact on the classification of independent restaurants featuring organic food. (RQ2)

H_{3o}: The profits from the operations of independent restaurants featuring organic food has no relationship with their classification. (RQ2)

H_{3a}: The profits from the operations of independent restaurants featuring organic food has a significant relationship with their classification. (RQ2)

Limitations and Delimitations

Independent restaurants that feature organic food are very limited to specific locations in metropolitan cities. Most restaurants in metropolitan cities tend to use local foods that in terms of price points are much lower in cost and much easier to obtain than ingredients for the preparation of organic food. When restaurant owners are searching for certified organic food ingredients, the list available to them tends to be limited. This makes the presence of restaurants that feature organic food few and far between, thereby making it difficult for researchers to collect necessary information for the proper conduct of empirical investigations. We contacted three of the major government agencies and an Organic Trade Association (FDA, USDA, and OTA) in the United States using various means—one being Facebook—and only two replied.

The researchers then used search engines and followed up with each restaurant to confirm if they in fact used enough organic food products to validate the research. In addition, part of the problem in researching this topic was that most of the independent restaurants involved in the industry find it difficult to share information about their business because the restaurant industry is very competitive. In the context of these challenges, the following limitations were identified as having the potential to restrict the generalizability of the research findings onto other situations:

1. The respondent may not be open to being truthful about their knowledge of organic produce. Many of the respondents may have mixed nonorganic or local ingredients with organic ones. Invariably, such a process may result in cross-contamination of "organic" and "local" food.
2. There may be many other factors, including availability due to price and seasonal availability, that affect organic food restaurants that the researcher may not have addressed.
3. The respondents may not have correctly calculated their profits consistent with other restaurants and average costs, thereby resulting in disparate data.
4. Because of the small sample size ($N = 36$), most independent restaurants in metropolitan cities in the United States were not included in the sample.

5. Members of the sample population might have been affected by their idiosyncratic and subjective views of the issues related to independent restaurants that feature organic foods in the United States.

6. Overall, the respondents may have refused to provide accurate information about their restaurants because of competitive pressures.

Delimitations

The delimitations constitute the boundaries set by this researcher to facilitate an effective interrogation of the research hypotheses and the results of the interaction of the dependent and independent variables. Thus, the delimitations that might affect the generalization of the research findings onto other situations are stated as follows:

1. The researchers understand that responding to surveys that are lengthy can be distracting, but the researcher requested respondents to complete as much as possible to aid in this study.

2. The researchers assume that the respondents provided accurate data. However, the researcher was unable to physically go to each city and meet with each restaurant owner to develop a rapport to assure the owners that the researcher had no other intentions besides using the data for dissertation research purposes.

3. A quantitative research approach that uses a large and randomized statistical sample size tends to yield more accurate results. However, one of the constraints of this study is the fact that the sample was purposively selected and that the sample size was relatively small with only ($N = 36$) participants.

4. Another delimitation of the study is the fact that the researchers were unable to obtain data on profits for more than one year.

Definitions of Terms

• Organic food: The term organic food as operationalized in this study refers to the organic food that preindustrial societies began cultivating in the agricultural stage. Organic food is naturally cultivated without any genetic modification production. Thus, the category of organic food is different from fruit and vegetables that do not include antibiotics and that trigger genetic and other biological or chemical modifications of food. Livestock such as chicken and cows must have access to the outdoors. Crops must not have been affected by synthetic modifications such as pesticides, petroleum-based fertilizers, bioengineered genes, and sewer sludge fertilizers that alter their processes of natural growth, composition, or taste (USDA, 2016).

- Independent restaurants: In terms of scale, independent restaurants are on a much smaller scale in comparison to their chain restaurant rivals. Independent restaurants are also owned and operated by their independent owner(s) and have the advantage of developing a brand and managing the loyalty of their customers by providing a quality experience and product. Because these operations tend to be nimble, their ability to be authentic and refine their products so that they cater to unique customers' needs and demands becomes much easier.

- Classification and types of restaurants: In *An Expanded Restaurant Typology*, Muller and Woods (1994) pointed out the distinct attributes and five categories of three restaurant segments. These categories are as follows: key to operation, customer decision, menu characteristics, strategic focus, and use of brand. Other authors have intimated that these characteristics and attributes are still present (Carvalho & Rodrigues, 2014). This researcher has applied three of the segments to this study. These segments are as follows:

  o Quick Service attributes:
     - Low price, speed, and consistency
     - Single-item focused/no customization/standard offerings
     - Self-service, process-driven technology
     - Market penetration and brand affiliation
     - Low price leadership

o   Midservice (family dining/coffee house):
  - Brand loyalty
  - Menu mix & choose, price and portion value
  - Table and counter service
  - Wide selection for menu option
  - Breakfast and lunch peak sales; food bars, buffets, and a la carte

o   Upscale Service (specializes in single cuisine, such as a steak house):
  - Unique name and product
  - Style, an experience
  - Customized, daily specials, high quality food

- Profits: Financial gains, especially the difference between the amount of revenue received and the amount spent in buying, operating, or producing something. Profits are further regarded as a valuable return. They are also the excess of returns over expenditures in a transaction or series of transactions. In effect, profits are an excess of a selling price of goods over their costs of production.

- Average cost: The construct of average cost was operationalized in this study as any cost that is equal to total cost divided by the number of goods (Q) produced. It is also equal to the sum of average variable costs plus average fixed costs (total fixed cost divided by quantity (Q). The diagram (Figure 1.1) below depicts a conceptual model that also encapsulates the critical stages of the doctoral dissertation research process. This process invariably includes the exploration and refinement of existing ideas through literature search, critical reading, and questioning, as well as the generation of research questions and hypotheses.

Figure 1.1 also shows the remaining stages of the research process that result in the reporting of findings that then leads to the beginning of new lines of research through more critical evaluation of an existing body of literature, in addition to the idiosyncratic experiences of the researcher, all in a loop fashion.

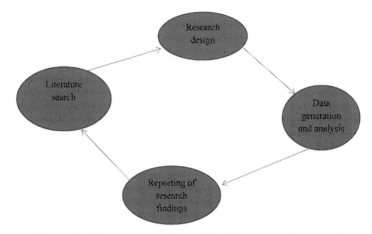

Figure 1.1. A conceptual model of the research process.

Summary and Conclusion

Figure 1.1 above identifies a conceptual model that also encapsulates the critical stages of this doctoral dissertation research process. One should note that the pattern is a continuous circle which provides direction for any future researcher to repeat the steps.

This chapter presented the problem background to this study in terms of the underlying reasons that led to the selection of this topic. The underlying research questions that served as guideposts to the study were provided. Similarly, the chapter provided the purpose and nature of this study. The statement of the problem was also encapsulated in this discussion. Next, the study presented the significance of the study and the research hypotheses. The limitations and delimitations of the study were also provided as well as the definitions of terms. It was posited that the central objective of this study was to provide some contributions to the survey literature in terms of the operations of three categories of independent restaurants that provide organic food on their menus.

Chapter Two
Literature Review

Introduction

This literature review chapter discusses prior empirical and theoretical studies that have focused on independent restaurants. The literature review examines two broad conceptual and theoretical perspectives that were used as a basis for this dissertation. The first focuses on the factors that determine the success and failure of independent restaurants. The second focuses on the influence of leadership factors on the organizational climate of independent restaurants, including those that feature organic food. This chapter also attempts to identify gaps in prior academic studies. We suggest that to a large extent, it was critical awareness of these gaps that informed the rationale for this study. The final section of this chapter focuses on the summary and conclusion.

Success and Failure of Restaurants

Angelo et al. (2008) examined the success factors for independent restaurant owners in the San Francisco Bay Area and concluded that internal factors, such as overconfidence and emotional unfitness, led to failure among these independent restaurants. The authors outlined variables that contribute to restaurant success. These included the following: strategic choices, competitive factors, marketing, resources, and capabilities. In a more recent study by Parsa et al. (2015), an essential ingredient for the success of independent restaurants was defined. Citing another author, Parsa et al. defined success as follows: "Success in business is defined in terms of rate of return on sales, and age or longevity of the firm" (p. 2).

Other studies, including one by Jennings and Beaver (as cited in Parsa et al., 2015), examined the "intangible goals of the small business owners in defining success" (p. 2). Success was also defined in this study as "the sustained satisfaction…and the attainment of certain pre-defined objectives which satisfy stakeholder aspirations" (Jennings and Beaver as cited in Parsa et al., 2015, p. 2).

There are factors that also account for the failure of independent restaurants (Parsa et al., 2005). However, Parsa et al. (2005) claimed that there is no universal definition of restaurant failure (p. 305). Thus, it is suggested that studies that use a "narrow definition of failure such as bankruptcy" tend to have the lowest failure rate, while those that focus on a broad definition, such as change of ownership, tend to have the highest failure rate. Parsa, Self, Sydnor-Busso, and Yoon (2011) suggested that organizational mortality in the restaurant sector could be based on restaurant location, affiliation, and/or size. The concept of affiliation is framed in this text as the presence of multiunit location of restaurants in a defined geographic space (Parsa et al., 2011, p. 360).

These are some of the factors the authors deemed as critical to understanding organizational failure from a population ecology perspective (Parsa et al., 2011, p. 360). Unlike the construct of rate of return on sales, as adopted by Parsa et al. (2014), the current study used profits among other variables to rank independent restaurants into three categories. This approach to gauging the success of the restaurants in the sample was used because the researcher could not gain access to information on rates of return. Thus, profits were used in this study as one of the many factors that define success. The three categories identified in the sample were: Quick Service, Midservice, and Upscale restaurants. Angelo et al. (2008) elaborated on the concept of the organizational life cycle, indicating that all organizations pass through certain stages in a life cycle. The authors noted:

> At any point along these life-cycle stages, a business can suffer setback catastrophic enough to lead to failure. Throughout the life cycle, the first stage is the most vulnerable, which is why the highest proportion of businesses that close are relatively new. "This liability of newness" has linked organizational adolescence

to increased organizational mortality rates. (Angelo et al., 2008, p. 306)

The authors also noted that one reason for early failure is that new businesses are typically not resource-endowed enough to allow them to become flexible or adapt to changing conditions. Building on the work of Kotler, Bowen, and Makens (1996), Angelo et al. (2008) discussed competitive factors as involving restaurant density or competitive intensity, knowledge of competitive forces, and product relevance.

Parsa et al. (2014) acknowledged that location is a significant factor in a restaurant's survival chances in a study based in Boulder, Colorado. The authors also noted that specific characteristics of Boulder, such as the city having a substantial population of apartment dwellers and transient residents (notably, university students), buttressed the restaurant's success.

The authors also suggested, in line with one of the current study's major hypotheses, that larger restaurants and those with a chain affiliation had a greater probability of success than small, Quick Service operations. The authors concluded that the factors that had a limited effect on a restaurant's success or failure were unemployment rates, the nature of nearby residents' profession, and the geographical presence of families with children under 18.

Dziadkowiec and Rood (2015) provided valuable insights into grasping some of the cultural differences among customers regarding preferences in casual dining service. The authors suggested that restaurant managers will be able to apply in their practices some of the ideas they offered to better understand differences between customers with cultural differences (p. 86). The authors also suggested that this study could form the basis for more extensive critical examination of the construct of cultural differences in the casual dining restaurant segment (p. 87). Mathe (2012) explored the relationship between unit food safety performance, labor costs, and revenues in Quick Service restaurants.

Mathe (2012) used a theoretical perspective that proposed organizational learning as a foundation for lowering labor costs (p. 398). The study found relationships among the variables, supporting the claim that lower labor costs typically result in greater financial and food safety performance. The study also concluded that greater food safety performance also tended to result in greater financial performance. Mathe posited that labor costs that are too high are essentially additional inputs that do not provide output that improves average costs (pp. 401-402). Commenting on the question of the relationship between excessive labor costs and profits and losses, the author intimated:

> Based on this logic, excessive labor costs should negatively influence profits and losses of the stores due to unnecessary employees on the clock. Similarly, excessive labor on the clock can create operational inefficiencies, with overcrowding in the facilities or flow through of the product being mishandled by too many people striving to finish the task in a timely manner. (p. 401)

Some studies have shown that failure to manage work and family life balance has been associated with restaurant failure (Camillo et al., 2008; Parsa et al., 2005). In a recent study by Agarwal and Dahm (2015), it was reported that assistance from family members played an important role in the operation of independent ethnic restaurants.

We hypothesized that it is possible that support from family members may also be a significant factor in the success of independent restaurants that feature organic food in metropolitan cities in the United States. The study by Agarwal and Dahm (2015) also found that culinary education and hospitality management background was ranked the least important factor that counted for success. The authors noted that this perception was surprising as most of the participants in this study were highly educated.

Agarwal and Dahm (2015) speculated that this ranking may have been due to the fact that 15 out of 20 survey participants had no educational background specific to the restaurant industry. Poulston and Yiu (2011) conducted research using a qualitative approach based on five semistructured interviews with Auckland restaurateurs offering organic menus. The authors concluded that while Upscale restaurants prioritized profits over principles, others prioritized their environmental beliefs. Poor support from the government, price premiums, and poor market demand were identified by participants in this study as obstacles to the development of organic dining in New Zealand.

Organizational Leadership and Culture

Organizational leadership and culture are vital tools that enhance organizational performance. In fact, a study conducted by Agarwal and Dahm (2015) concluded that ethnic restaurant owners embraced the notion that competent management was the most important contributor to success. Several studies have emphasized the critical ingredients that instigate organizational success in the independent segment of the restaurant industry (Angelo et al., 2008; Bayou & Bennett, 1992; Bertsimas & Shioda, 2003; Parsa, 2005).

We note that these critical ingredients are also imperative for organic independent restaurants. Angelo et al. (2008) discussed some of the critical factors that affect the failure rate of independent restaurants. The authors developed a restaurant viability model that identified family life cycle, organizational life cycle, and internal and external processes as determinants of restaurant viability. These observations are in line with those made by Parsa et al. (2005), who argued that past research on restaurant failures focused mainly on quantitative factors, ignoring other important qualitative factors such as the nature of organizational leadership (p. 369).

This perspective tended to be buttressed by authors like Keasey and Watson (as cited in Parsa et al., 2005, p. 369) who have suggested that traditional financial models may not be appropriate for making a comprehensive assessment of the viability of new and small ventures. These assumptions lead to one important fact: Leadership is a critically important variable in terms of the underlying factors that account for organizational success. Cichy, Sciarini, and Patton (1992) enumerated four areas of competency that leaders should possess: attention through vision, meaning through communication, trust through positioning, and the development of self through positive self-regard (p. 48). Leaders are expected to be able to create a sense of outcome that draws others in and encourages them to become similarly committed (Cichy et al., 1992, p. 48).

Leaders are also able to communicate their sense of vision with clarity and purpose (Cichy et al., 1992, p. 48). Further, the authors noted that leaders should be required to consistently demonstrate and earn trust through their reliability, predictability, and accountability (Cichy et al., 1992, p. 48). Similarly, the authors noted that inconsistency breeds misunderstanding and distrust, which are obstacles that are not easily overcome (Cichy et al., 1992, p. 48). Effective leaders are also perceived as ones who know their strengths and consistently work to enhance them (Cichy et al., 1992, p. 48). In addition, leaders typically recognize their shortcomings and seek to compensate for them (Cichy et al., 1992, p. 48). It is suggested that the capacity to improve upon their skills is what distinguishes "leaders" from "followers" (Cichy et al., 1992, p. 48).

Gill et al. (2011) posited that the importance of retaining staff cannot be ignored. Indeed, it was also suggested that transformational leadership has a direct impact on the empowerment of employees and their willingness to quit. These authors examined the impact of many different factors on employee intention to quit, which in turn leads to high employee turnover. The authors further posited that high employee turnover is not in the favor of service organizations like independent restaurants because it has a direct impact on hiring and training costs. These perspectives line up with some of the findings of the current research. Thus, as discussed above, the willingness of restaurant owners to exhibit responsibility and honesty and to encourage further training for their employees could be perceived as some of the effective leadership strategies required for the success of their restaurants.

Another important aspect of transformational and effective leadership is the organizational culture that leaders, be they owners of independent or chain restaurants, can help create in the organization. Gill et al. (2011) stressed the importance of retaining staff. In this study, a negative relationship was found between (a) employee-perceived empowerment and employee-perceived intention to quit and (b) employee-perceived transformational leadership used by managers and employee intention to quit. This study made several recommendations to managers and owners of hospitality organizations for improving employee retention and for reducing intentions to quit.

Clement (1994) suggested that research should focus on an organization's culture in order to concentrate on organizational practices rather than values. This idea was borrowed from studies conducted by Verbeke (2000) who extensively studied organizational culture and its dimensions. Writing about how an organizational culture encourages innovation and change, Boisnier and Chatman (2002) defined the concept of organizational culture as follows:

> A good way to grasp the concept of company culture is to think of a firm as a mini-civilization. All civilizations have a group of animating beliefs and values that gives meaning, purpose, and direction. These beliefs constitute culture. The United States, for example, is centered on the beliefs and values found in the Declaration of Independence and our Constitution. If you reduce those beliefs down to their essence, you might say that our national animating principles are "equality before the law," "life, liberty and the pursuit of happiness," among others. (pp. 121-122)

Boisnier and Chatman (2002) further suggested that culture is an essential ingredient for organizational success because it offers a sense of permanence, direction, and marketplace identity, and also helps us find our natural allies (pp. 123-134). Roxborough (2000) suggested that organizational culture is critically important to fostering the debates that are necessary for successful innovation within the organization. Kaarst et al. (2004) researched the organizational cultures of libraries and concluded that organizational culture is a strategic resource that must be harnessed. Organizational culture can also be a basis for legitimacy-seeking as suggested by institutional theory (Dickson, BeShears, & Gupta, 2004).

Goldman (1993) conducted research on the concept selection for independent restaurants and concluded that for independent restaurants to thrive, they must have a clear-cut identity and a defined concept that caters to a specific group. Ogbeide and Harrington (2011) conducted research on management in the food service industry and concluded that larger organizational structure requires higher levels of involvement by middle and lower management levels to successfully make use of strategic processes.

The authors further suggested that food service firms in their study adopted a similar participative management style for larger or smaller food service firms (Ogbeide & Harrington, 2011, p. 733). In a study of Quick Service restaurants, DiPietro and Strate (2006) found that the positive perception held by managers with respect to older workers did not translate into a stated desire to actually hire a larger percentage of older workers to staff the restaurants. Cumberland and Herd (2011) viewed the culture of the organization as a tool for determining which interventions may be appropriate during a merger, acquisition, or divestiture. The authors noted the importance of the study of organizational culture in small franchise restaurants and other restaurant types as well.

Gaps in Prior Academic Studies

Upon careful and critical examination of the extant literature, this researcher has observed several gaps in current empirical studies that have informed the rationale of the current study. Thus, areas that constitute gaps in the literature are the lack of empirical studies of profits and costs to examine the health of an organization. Thus, this researcher suggests that future studies should focus on obtaining time series data on costs and profits that reflect a longer time horizon, perhaps five years or more. It is doubtless that such data might yield more accurate results. We further suggest that future research should not focus solely on independent restaurants that feature organic food in general, but independent ethic restaurants that also feature organic food in metropolitan cities in the United States as well.

This recommendation follows from the realization informed by the available data that there are many ethnic independent restaurants that are involved in the organic food business. And yet, empirical studies on this topic are difficult to find. In a recent study on ethnic restaurants, Agarwal and Dahm (2015) indicated that the number and popularity of ethnic restaurants have increased dramatically. It was suggested that in 1980, ethnic restaurants amounted to only 10% of all restaurants, but by 2001, they constituted 23% (Agarwal & Dahm, 2015; Roseman, 2006). It was further intimated that the demand for ethnic food from a burgeoning immigrant population has spurred growth in the number of ethnic restaurants. Agarwal and Dahm (2015) noted that researchers have identified factors that contribute to overall restaurant success; however, they concluded it is uncertain whether these factors affect independent ethnic restaurants in the same way.

As previously noted, empirical studies on independent organic restaurants are few and far between. We call for more comparative research that focuses on making cross-country comparisons. The aim of such efforts would be to examine both managers' and customers' perceptions about issues of sustainability, concerns about the environment, healthy foods, and animal rights activities around the world and how these affect menu choices. In addition, it would be beneficial to determine how the entrepreneurial spirit is galvanized to respond to these choices.

Summary and Conclusion

This literature review chapter discussed current empirical and theoretical studies that have focused on independent restaurants. The success and failure of restaurants has been discussed in some detail. This chapter has also critically examined leadership factors that influence the organizational climate of independent restaurants, including organic independent restaurants. The chapter pointed out the gaps in current empirical studies and suggested that to a large extent, it is critical awareness of these gaps that informed the rationale for this study.

In the final chapter of this dissertation, we called for various ways the existing literature on independent organic restaurants could be enhanced. We also called for diversifying the scope of research by conducting empirical and theoretical studies on independent ethnic restaurants that feature organic food in metropolitan cities in the United States. It is suggested that one of the rationales for this call is the fact that many regions of the world are experiencing high growth rates in the consumption of organic foods (Poulston & Yiu, 2011). Further, the perceived health benefits are expected to dominate consumers' preferences for organic food in the future (Poulston & Yiu, 2011, p. 185).

Chapter Three
Methodology

Introduction

In Chapter One, we discussed the problem background in terms of the underlying reasons that led to the selection of the research topic and the importance of this study. The limitations and delimitations of the study were also provided as well as the definition of terms. In Chapter Two, the body of research literature that undergirded this study was critically reviewed. The chapter also critically examined leadership factors that lead to the success of independent restaurants. In addition, the chapter called for various ways the current literature on independent organic restaurants could be enhanced. We also called for diversifying the scope of research by conducting empirical and theoretical studies on independent ethnic restaurants that feature organic foods in metropolitan cities in the United States.

The current chapter presents the methodological framework that has undergirded this study. It also presents a restatement of the research problem. The chapter further discusses the research design, including the characteristics and type of survey instrument adopted. The methodological assumptions that ensured validity of the research findings are also posited. The chapter presents the selection of the research participants as well as data analysis. Furthermore, the chapter also discusses the validity and reliability of the study. In addition, the ethical considerations that were the guideposts for this study are presented.

The Five-Step Hypothesis Testing Procedure

Due to the nature of testing hypotheses, the researchers were not able to survey all independent restaurant owners/managers featuring organic food within the United States. Hence, a nonrandom sample ($N = 36$) was selected to represent this particular population. The null and alternative hypotheses were formulated and tested on the basis of data that reflected the parameters of this sample (Creswell, 2003, 2009; Field, 2009). As part of the five-step hypothesis testing procedure, the null and alternative hypotheses are stated.

Statement of the Null and Alternative Hypotheses

H_{1o}: The average cost associated with the sale of each meal has no impact on the classification of independent restaurants featuring organic food.

H_{1a}: The average cost associated with the sale of each meal has an impact on the classification of independent restaurants featuring organic food.

H_{2o}: The average cost associated with the sale of each meal has no impact on the days of operation of independent restaurants featuring organic food.

H_{2a}: The average cost associated with the sale of each meal has a significant impact on the days of operation of independent restaurants featuring organic food.

H_{3o}: The profits from the operations of independent restaurants featuring organic food have no relationship with their classification.

H_{3a}: The profits from the operations of independent restaurants featuring organic food have a significant relationship with their classification.

H_{4o}: The life cycle of independent restaurants featuring organic food has no impact on their profits.

H_{4a}: The life cycle of independent restaurants featuring organic food has a significant impact on their profits.

Statement of the Appropriate Test Static and Level of Significance

Both correlation and regression analyses were used to test the null hypotheses. The researcher chose a level of significance of $p < .05$ for the correlation analysis and a level of significance of $p < .01$ for the stepwise regression analysis. The aim of this analytical strategy was to ensure quality insurance such as increasing the accuracy and robustness of the results of the linear stepwise regression model.

Statement of the Decision Rules

The decision rules the researcher adhered to in this study suggested that the null hypotheses would be accepted if the results showed a significance level of $p < .05$. On the other hand, if the results showed a significance level of $p > .05$, then the null hypothesis would be rejected. The four null hypotheses were used to address the following two essential research questions:

1. To what extent do factors such as the average cost associated with the sale of each meal, profits, and life cycle influence independent restaurants that feature organic foods in metropolitan cities in the United States?

2. To what extent do average cost associated with the sale of each meal and profit influence the classification of independent restaurants that feature organic foods in metropolitan cities in the United States into Quick Service, Midservice, and Upscale?

Computing the Appropriate Test Statistic

This step presupposes that when the values are computed, the researcher must either reject or accept the null hypothesis. In the case of the first research question (RQ1) stipulated for this study, the following null hypotheses were accepted:

H_{2a}: The average cost associated with the sale of each meal has a significant impact on the days of operation of independent restaurants featuring organic foods.

H_{4o}: The life cycle of independent restaurants featuring organic food has no impact on their profits.

In the case of the second research question (RQ2), the following alternative hypotheses were accepted:

H_{1a}: The average cost associated with the sale of each meal has an impact on the classification of independent restaurants featuring organic food.

H_{3a}: The profits from the operations of independent restaurants featuring organic food have a significant relationship with their classification.

Interpretation of the Decision

The results of hypothesis testing on the four stipulated null hypotheses revealed several findings. First, the findings showed that average cost associated with the sale of each organic meal was highly correlated with the number of days the restaurants were opened. Similarly, the stage the restaurants were at in their maturation process (life cycle) had no statistically significant relationship with the profits earned by the independent restaurants in the sample during the fiscal period of 2015. Further findings revealed that average cost had an impact on classification, profits had a significant relationship with classification, and life cycle had an impact on profits, while average cost had an impact on the amount of days the restaurants were operating.

Methodology

In this chapter, the researchers will investigate the impact of the independent variables on the dependent variables in regards to determining the factors that influence the preferences of independent restaurant owners that feature organic foods in metropolitan cities ranging in population size from 1,197,800 to 3,792,700, rounding to the nearest hundred. The researcher targeted 10 cities due to the popularity of organic foods restaurants in these regions in the United States. These cities included Chicago, Atlanta, Dallas, Los Angeles, Nashville, New York City, Portland, Seattle, Denver, and Washington. Prior studies (see Parsa et al., 2011) suggested that independent restaurants have pointed to the fact that independent restaurants endure a higher rate of failure during their initial years of operation. For small restaurants and niche independents restaurants, it can be even more challenging to survive the travails of stiff competition.

Prior studies have suggested that independent business owners play the most important role in the success or failure of a business, even when featuring organic foods (Gon & Kim, 2004; Poulston & Yiu, 2011). The researchers examined this phenomenon by surveying random organic independent restaurant owners. The methodology for this study was quantitative. Obtaining information about a host of variables in order to render accurate assessments of the restaurants in the sample was the major objective of the research process.

Another critical objective of designing this study was to ensure that the methodology and statistical models chosen for analyses actually fit the data collected (Creswell, 2014). The literature on research methodology indicates that there are three types of methodologies a researcher could consider: qualitative, quantitative, and mixed methods. According to Creswell, qualitative research is an approach geared at exploring patterns and trends and understanding behaviors and attitudes. Quantitative research, on the other hand, relies on identifying variables and constructing hypotheses about the relationship between them (Camillo et al., 2008).

Thus, quantitative research uses variables to measure or observe an event, and as a result, seeks to determine how one variable affects another. The types of variables are: independent, dependent, intervening or meditating, moderating, control, and confounding (Creswell, 2014). To determine which variables are used for research, a theory is constructed to establish an argument or rationale, or to even assist in explaining or predicting a phenomenon (Creswell, 2014).

Restatement of the Research Problem

As stated in Chapter One, one of the problems that provided the rationale for this research is the current paucity of data on the organic food business. Given the current state of affairs in the food and hospitality industry, one is led to believe that organic food is being purchased on a relatively large scale, which is why there may be limited survey research investigating the pattern of demand in this sector. Chapter One recognized that consumers today are taking more care to know where their food comes from and what is in that food. However, the problem is that little research has been conducted to investigate the variables that affect the current pattern of demand for organic foods, let alone how independent restaurants are positioning themselves to furnish the need in this market (Budhwar, 2004).

Because of the aforementioned challenges, the researcher noted that gathering data on this particular subject is an uphill task (Budhwar, 2004). One should recognize the fact that those consumers who are health and nutrition conscious possess necessary awareness and knowledge of food and labels. However, for those consumers who are not health conscious, labels may not have an effect when selecting a lower calorie item from the menu (Ellison, 2013).

Chapter One also recognized the fact that because of these and other reasons, a study of this nature to serve as a breach and fill in some of these gaps in scholarly and popular knowledge, information and understanding could not be more relevant at this current point in time. As it was indicated in chapter one, this research problem has given rise to the research questions and hypotheses stated in the subsequent section

Restatement of the Research Questions and Hypotheses

The following research questions were stipulated to structure and guide the research process:

1. To what extent do factors such as the average cost associated with the sale of each meal, profits, and life cycle influence independent restaurants that feature organic foods in metropolitan cities in the United States?
2. To what extent do average cost associated with the sale of each meal and profits influence the classification of independent restaurants that feature organic food in metropolitan cities in the United States into Quick Service, Midservice, and Upscale?

Restatement of Research Hypotheses

The four research hypotheses that guided this study are restated here as follows:

H_{1o}: The average cost associated with the sale of each meal has no impact on the classification of independent restaurants featuring organic food.

H_{1a}: The average cost associated with the sale of each meal has an impact on the classification of independent restaurants featuring organic food.

H_{2o}: The average cost associated with the sale of each meal has no impact on the days of operation of independent restaurants featuring organic food.

H_{2a}: The average cost associated with the sale of each meal has a significant impact on the days of operation of independent restaurants featuring organic food.

H_{3o}:   The profits from the operations of independent restaurants featuring organic food have no relationship with their classification.

H_{3a}:   The profits from the operations of independent restaurants featuring organic food have a significant relationship with their classification.

H_{4o}:   The life cycle of independent restaurants featuring organic food has no impact on their profits.

H_{4a}:   The life cycle of independent restaurants featuring organic food has a significant impact on their profits.

Research Design

This study utilized a quantitative survey approach. The intended purpose of this methodology was to highlight some of the features of the three categories of restaurants identified in the sample ($N = 36$). The data generated were analyzed using correlation and regression analysis. A one-way ANOVA test was also performed on the data. The aim of using a one-way ANOVA test was to compare the mean average cost per menu of the three groups of independent restaurants that feature organic foods in the metropolitan cities in the United States that appeared in the sample ($N = 36$). Although the tests helped to determine the strength of the relationship between two variables, they could not predict 100% causality.

Procedures

The researchers used self-administered surveys to collect data for this research. The surveys were distributed on the basis of a purposive or convenience sampling involving independent restaurant owners. The researchers utilized two attempts to obtain the data used in this research. The first attempt was made through the use of a third party called Sendit Media. No response was yielded through this approach. Hence, a second attempt was made by the researcher Watson et al. (2008) indicated using online software is a platform where communities sharing their experience and so the researchers used the application named Yelp. We used Yelp to obtain information about the perceptions of potential restaurant owners and managers (research participants) throughout 10 metropolitan cities in the United States. The mode of communication with potential research participants was email accessed through the websites of listed independent restaurant owners that agreed to participate in this study.

One hundred questionnaires were sent out to the potential research participants. However, only 36 participants completed the surveys. This amounted to about 36% of the expected responses. The invitation to participate in the research study was done through a letter (see Appendix 1) that informed the potential participants about the study and asked them to voluntarily participate in the survey.

The length of the questionnaire was moderate and participants were expected to complete the survey in 20 min or less. Consequently, this researcher expected a low nonresponse rate and assumed that most potential participants would respond to the survey. The participants remained anonymous. A response rate of 36 out of 100 questionnaires sent out to potential respondents was somewhat consistent with the researcher's expectations.

Methodological Assumptions

The current study involved a quantitative research design. Like other methodological approaches, a quantitative survey design of this type has several assumptions. They could be stipulated as follows:

1. The participants in the survey were owners of independent restaurants interested in the topic of organic foods.
2. The survey instrument constructed for this study was applicable for the design of the study and the purpose for which it was used.
3. The responses given by the respondents in the study reflected the truth.
4. Our impact on the data collected was not significant and should not be considered as a factor in the findings of this study.

Selection of Participants

Surveys were distributed among 100 independent restaurants in 10 metropolitan cities that had more than 30 organic food restaurants. The selection of the locations was purposeful due to the congregation of organic restaurants. In each metropolitan city, there was an average of 10 organic restaurants providing more than just one organic item. The sample was determined using purposive nonrandom sampling techniques. Due to the lack of resources, it was much more convenient for the researcher to use a purposive approach to gather the data. The cities used were indicated by zip code and no business names were used in this research. The independent restaurants that were targeted were those that indicated the word *organic* on their menus.

These restaurants can be classified under the categories of Quick Service, Midservice, and Upscale. Only the owners of the restaurants in the sample were targeted for this study. The questionnaire was sent by email to potential participants in the study. The potential participants were instructed through a consent form sent to them via email that they had the complete freedom to choose to participate or not in the study. The responses were sent back to the researcher through email.

The featured organic foods ranged from organic condiments, casual sandwiches, and cold-pressed juices to vegan meat substitutes to upscale entrees serving high-end cuisine using high-quality products. The expectation of this researcher was that respondents met the two essential criteria: (a) their restaurants must have been in operation for more than five years and (b) they must be classified as independent restaurants that serve organic foods.

Instrumentation

Both the independent and dependent variables were determined or measured using items on the administered survey. There was a battery of 37 questions or items (see Appendix 3). The responses were a variation of the typical 5-point Likert scale (i.e., Poor-1, Fair-2, Average-3, Good-4, Excellent-5; see Appendix 3), dichotomous questions requiring yes or no responses, multiple choice questions requiring choices to be made from a limited amount of options (one out of six choices), and an unstructured open-ended question allowing the respondent to add any additional information.

One of the most important objectives of the survey was to provide responses to the essential research questions. Another important objective of the survey was to measure the relative success or failure of independent restaurants that feature foods in different segments of restaurants: Quick Service, Midscale, and Upscale. In constructing the survey instrument for this study, questionnaires were adapted and modified from several previous studies (Camillo et al., 2008; Inwood, 2004, 2009; Parsa et al., 2005).

Data Collection and Analysis

Various forms of data collection techniques were used to generate data for this study. However, the primary mode of data collection which led to the generation of primary data was the administration of a survey instrument. The survey data were coded to facilitate analysis. Furthermore, the Statistical Package for the Social Sciences (SPSS) software was used to analyze the data. The researchers used descriptive statistics as well as inferential statistics to analyze the data and make inferences about the sample population. Several null hypotheses were formulated to test the degree of associations between the dependent and independent variables. Regression analysis was also used. Data for this study were collected both by electronic (email) responses and hard copy.

Validity and Reliability of the Survey Results

Both dependent and independent variables were used in the study. Three statistical tests, correlation analysis, regression, and a one-way ANOVA were utilized in order to understand the degree of interaction between variables that were designated dependent and those that were designated independent. Dependent variables tend to derive their values from the independent variables, especially when using regression models (Creswell, 2003).

In a classic study on the successes and failures of restaurants, two known researchers, Parsa (2005) and Camillo (2008), used a combination of qualitative and quantitative methods. To attain the highest level of reliability and validity, a questionnaire in combination with interviews were utilized. Previous sections of this chapter focused on a restatement of the research problem. They also focused on research design, instrumentation, methodological assumptions, and so forth.

Ethical Considerations

The invitation to participate in the research study was done through a consent letter that informed the potential participants about the study and asked them to voluntarily participate in the survey. Participants of the study also remained anonymous throughout the study. Thus, no physical or psychological coercion was used in this study. These efforts were geared at fulfilling the fundamental precepts of ethical research embodied in the literature on research ethics. They were also consistent with the suggestions offered by Mill and Weber and other authors (see Halse, 2005).

The Mill and Weber tradition instructs us that ethical social science must insist that research subjects have the right to be informed about the nature and consequences of experiments in which they are involved (Halse, 2005, p. 144). There are two necessary ethical requirements that researchers must meet in recruiting subjects to participate in their experiments: First, subjects must agree voluntarily to participate without physical and psychological coercion. Second, the agreement of subjects must be based on full and open information.

These cardinal principles are also enshrined in the Articles of the Nuremburg Tribunal and the Declaration of Helsinki. These ethical codes of conduct that should guide any ethical research project state that subjects must be informed about the duration, methods, possible risks, and the purpose or aim of the experiment (Halse, 2005, p. 144). Under the terms of the Belmont Report, researchers are encouraged to ensure that researchers enter the research voluntarily and receive adequate information about the procedures and possible consequences of the experiments. The principle of beneficence stipulates that researchers should do everything they can to secure the well-being of their subjects. Beneficent actions are discussed under the terms of the Belmont Report as follows:

> In the case of particular projects, investigators and members of their institutions are obliged to give forethought to the maximization of benefits and the reduction of risks that might occur from the research investigation. In the case of scientific research in general, members of the larger society is obliged to recognize the larger term benefits and risks that may result from the improvement of knowledge and from the development of novel medical, psychotherapeutic, and social procedures. (University of Illinois at Urbana-Champaign as cited in Hales, 2005, p. 146)

Merriam (2002) intimated that a good qualitative study must be one that has been carried out in an ethical manner. In addition, Merriam indicated that the validity and reliability of a study depend upon the ethics of the researcher. This researcher recognizes the fact that these statements are instructive for quantitative researchers as well. Indeed, this researcher should note that the ethical standards set by researchers conducting research in the quantitative tradition in terms of how subjects or participants are treated can have a profound effect on the validity and reliability of quantitative research findings.

It is for this reason that government agencies in various countries around the world have insisted that the review and monitoring of entities be set up by institutions engaged in research involving human subjects. Institutional review boards (IRBs) embody the utilitarian agenda in terms of assumptions, scope, and a procedural guideline (Hales, 2005, p. 146). The United States National Commission for the Protection of Human Subjects in Biomedical and Behavioral Research was established in 1976. As the result of establishing this institution, the three principles alluded to above were established: respect for persons, beneficence, and justice.

Summary and Conclusion

This chapter presented the methodological framework that undergirded this study. It also presented a restatement of the research problem. The chapter further discussed the research design, including the characteristics and type of survey instrument adopted. The methodological assumptions that ensured validity of the research findings were also established. The chapter presented the selection of the research participants as well as data analysis. Furthermore, the chapter discussed the validity and reliability of the study. In addition, the ethical considerations that were the guideposts for this study were discussed in this chapter.

Chapter Four
Results

Introduction

In Chapter One, the researcher discussed the problem background in terms of the underlying reasons that led to the selection of the research topic. The limitations and delimitations of the study were also provided as well as the definitions of terms. In Chapter Two, the body of research literature that undergirded this study was critically reviewed. In Chapter Three, we critically examined leadership factors that influence the organizational climate of independent restaurants, including those that feature organic foods.

We also called for diversifying the scope of research by conducting empirical and theoretical studies on independent ethnic restaurants that feature organic foods in metropolitan cities in the United States. In this chapter, we will provide results of the data analysis and a restatement of the research purpose in an attempt to respond to the research questions and hypotheses. Descriptive statistics are also presented on the dependent and independent variables.

We noted it was primarily through the review of pertinent aspects of the existing body of literature on restaurants featuring organic foods and prior lived experiences of the researcher that gave form and content to the research questions and hypotheses. Prior chapters in this dissertation also presented the research methodology and design. It is suggested that a survey approach was adopted to explore and provide clues to the research problem, question, and null hypotheses. This chapter provides the results of the data analysis in an attempt to explain some of the factors that affect independent restaurants that feature organic foods in the United

States. Descriptive statistics as well as inferential statistics are provided and analyzed in this chapter.

Restatement of the Research Purpose

The primary purpose of this study was to conduct an analysis of independent restaurants featuring organic food in the United States. This study was conducted within the framework of a quantitative approach, involving adult participants ranging in ages of 21 to 51-plus. The data were collected through the use of a survey to investigate how each of the participants' demographic characteristics and other variables such as profits, education, qualifications of restaurant owners, years of operation, and average cost impacted restaurant classifications. The survey instrument was influenced by a basic 5-point Likert-type scale, drawing on prior scales constructed by Bagby, Taylor, and Parker (1992) and Camillo et al. (2008).

The study also investigated how average cost of an item on the menu impacted the days of operation of independent restaurants featuring organic foods. Similarly, the study further investigated how the life cycle of organic restaurants impacted their profits and average cost of an item on the menu. The various ways in which survey participants viewed their own leadership traits were also probed—using risk-taking as a proxy—to examine how they were influenced by other variables, such as average cost of an item on the menu, amount of training employees received, honesty, as well as the number of customers served per week.

Descriptive Statistics

This section will present descriptive statistics for the continuous and categorical variables. It is suggested that while some of the variables have been classified as independent, others have been classified as dependent. Some of the variables, such as restaurant profits from selling organic foods, were classified both as dependent and independent variables in order to draw appropriate statistical inferences through performing both correlation and regression analyses on the data. Variables such as gender, age, training, education, and qualifications were extracted from the democratic section of the survey instrument.

Table 1.1

Descriptive Statistics for the Continuous Variables (N = 36)

Variables	Minimum	Maximum	Mean	SD
Age	1	3	1.67	.75
Education	2	6	4.17	.16
Average cost	1	3	3.00	.67
Distance	1	4	1.97	.81
Days of opera.	1	5	3.28	1.71
Finance	1	4	2.22	.89
Seating	2	2	2.00	.000
Training	1	4	3.03	1.11
Employees	1	4	3.22	.76
Menu changes	1	3	2.50	.81
Thoughts	1	4	1.83	.12
Profits	1	3	1.61	.80
Customers served per week	1	5	2.86	.80

Table 1.2

Descriptive Statistics for the Categorical Variables (N = 36)

Variables	Minimum	Maximum	Mean	SD
Gender	1	3	1.94	.86
Location	1	4	3.17	.77
Classification	1	3	2.00	.82
Life Cycle	2	3	2.11	.31
Emotionally Attached	1	1	1.00	.00
Advertisement	1	4	3.33	.47
Menu Category	1	6	5.33	1.63
Drive through	1	4	3.03	.12
Leadership traits	1	3	1.78	.48

Both categorical and continuous variables provided in the tables above were coded to facilitate analysis using the Statistical Package for the Social Sciences (SPSS). The keys can be found in Appendix 1.1. Tables 1.1 and 1.2 showed that there were a total of $(N = 36)$ individuals who participated in the survey. The categorical variable gender was coded with 1 designated for males, 2 designated for females, and 3 designated for both male and female owners (*SD* = .86). Thus, there were 14 male owners that constituted 38.9% of owners, 10 female owners that constituted about 27.8% of owners, and 12 mixed owners comprised of male and female owners. This figure constituted about 33.3% of owners of independent restaurants in the overall survey sample (*N* = 36).

The educational background of those who participated in the survey as shown in Table 1.1 above ranged from those who had less than a high school diploma to those who held a graduate degree. The average educational level of research participants was an associate degree. A total of 5.6% of survey participants had a high school diploma, 19.4% had some college but no degree, 30.6% had an associate degree, 41.7% had a bachelor's degree, and 2.8% had a graduate degree.

The qualifications of survey participants ranged from those who held degrees or certificates in hospitality to those who had no qualifications related to the restaurant business. This number constituted 5.6% of the total. The profits made by the various categories of restaurants in the sample ranged from $80,000 to $300,000 (*SD* = .80). Meanwhile, customers served per week ranged from between 100 and 300 to 1,001 and above (*SD* = .60). While three respondents stated that their restaurants were opened per week 8.3% of the time, 17 respondents stated that their restaurants were opened per week 47.2% of the time. Meanwhile, 16 respondents said that their restaurants were opened per week 44.4% of the time.

Restatement of the Research Questions and Hypotheses

This section lists the research questions and hypotheses of the study. As stated in Chapter One, there were two primary research questions and four null hypotheses the researcher framed for investigation in this study. Thus, the primary research questions that directed this study are restated here.

Restatement of Research Questions

The following research questions were stipulated to structure and guide the research process:

1. To what extent do factors such as the average cost associated with the sale of each meal, profits, and life cycle influence independent

restaurants that feature organic foods in metropolitan cities in the United States?

2. To what extent do average cost associated with the sale of each meal and profits influence the classification of independent restaurants that feature organic foods in metropolitan cities in the United States into Quick Service, Midservice, and Upscale?

Restatement of Research Hypotheses

The four research hypotheses that guided this study are restated here as follows:

H_{1o}: The average cost associated with the sale of each meal has no impact on the classification of independent restaurants featuring organic food.

H_{1a}: The average cost associated with the sale of each meal has an impact on the classification of independent restaurants featuring organic food.

H_{2o}: The average cost associated with the sale of each meal has no impact on the days of operation of independent restaurants featuring organic food.

H_{2a}: The average cost associated with the sale of each meal has a significant impact on the days of operation of independent restaurants featuring organic food.

H_{3o}: The profits from the operations of independent restaurants featuring organic food have no relationship with their classification.

H_{3a}: The profits from the operations of independent restaurants featuring organic food have a significant relationship with their classification.

H_{4o}: The life cycle of independent restaurants featuring organic food has no impact on their profits.

H_{4a}: The life cycle of independent restaurants featuring organic food has a significant impact on their profits.

Quantitative Results

Table 1.3

Correlation Analysis: Continuous and Categorical Predictor Variables on Classification

	r	p
Average cost	.663	.000**
Life cycle	.433	.008**
Days of operation	.402	.015*
Profits	.387	.020*

p<. 05* p< .01**

The results of the correlation analysis in Table 1.3 above show that there was a statistically significant relationship between average cost of an item on the menu and the classification of independent restaurants into Quick Service, Midservice, and Upscale as represented in the survey data (r = .663, p = .000). Consistent with what has been reported in Chapter Four, these findings demonstrate that the first null hypothesis was rejected while the alternative hypothesis was accepted. The findings also helped to address the first research question. This suggests that perhaps the three categories of restaurants were highly correlated (p < .01) with the average cost associated with services rendered at these restaurants. The results in the table above also show there was a statistically significant relationship between the stage at which the restaurants were at in terms of their life cycle (introduction, growing, maturity, decline) and the categories in which they belonged (r = .433, p = .008).

Furthermore, the number of days the restaurants were opened per week was correlated with the categories in which they were classified (r = .402, p = .015). The results in Table 1.3 above also show that there was a statistically significant relationship between profits and the classification of the restaurants into Quick Service, Midservice, and Upscale as represented by the survey participants (r = .387, p = .020).

Table 1.4

Correlation Analysis: Continuous and Categorical Predictor Variables on Days of Operation

	r	p
Classification	.402	.015*
Average cost	.663	.000**
Profits	.442	.007**

$p < .05^*, p < .01^{**}$

The results of the correlation analysis in Table 1.4 above show that there was a statistically significant relationship between the classification of independent restaurants into Quick Service, Midservice, and Upscale as represented in the survey data ($r = .015$, $p = .402$) and the number of days the restaurants were opened per week. Readers should note, however, that in as much as these findings reject the stipulated null hypotheses, they shed an important light on the analysis of factors that shape the success or failure of independent restaurants that feature organic foods in metropolitan cities in the United States.

This suggests that perhaps the three categories of restaurants were highly correlated ($p < .01$) with the number of days organic foods were sold at these restaurants. The results in the table above also show there was a statistically significant relationship between the average cost of an item on the menu and the number of days the restaurants were opened ($r = .663$, $p = .000$). Furthermore, there was a statistically significant relationship between the amount of profits accrued and the number of days the restaurants were opened ($r = .007$, $p = .442$).

Table 1.5

Correlation Analysis: Continuous and Categorical Predictor Variables on Profits

	r	p
Seating	-.378	.023*
Qualifications	.342	.041*
Education	.359	.031*
Honesty	-.404	.015*
Days of operation	.442	.007**

$p < .05*, p < .01**$

The results of the correlation analysis in Table 1.5 above show that there was a statistically significant relationship between the classification of independent restaurants into Quick Service, Midservice, and Upscale as represented on the survey data ($r = .015$, $p = .402$) and the number of days the restaurants were opened per week. As indicated above, these findings reject the stipulated null hypotheses. However, they shed an important light on the analysis of factors that shape the success or failure of independent restaurants that feature organic foods in metropolitan cities in the United States.

This suggests that perhaps the three categories of restaurants were highly correlated ($p < .01$) with the number of days they had organic foods on the menu. The results in the table above also showed there was statistically significant relationship between the average cost of an item on the menu and the number of days the restaurants were opened ($r = .663$, $p = .000$). Furthermore, there was a statistically significant relationship between the amount of profits accrued and the number of days the restaurants were opened ($r = .007$, $p = .442$). Thus, this result suggests that the volume of sales was closely linked to profits.

Table 1.6

Correlation Analysis: Continuous and Categorical Predictor Variables on Leadership Traits

	r	p
Average cost	.349	.037*
Customers served per week	-.336	.045*
Training	.384	.021*
Responsibility	.386	.020*
Honesty	.368	.027*
Life Cycle	.229	-.205

$p < .05^*$, $p < .01^{**}$

The results of Table 1.6 above show that seating had a statistically significant relationship with profits ($r = -.378$, $p = .023$). The qualifications of the restaurant owners also had a statistically significant relationship with profits ($r = .342$, $p = .041$). These findings reject the stipulated null hypotheses. The results of hypotheses testing are reported and discussed in Chapter Four. However, readers should note that they shed an important light on the analysis of factors that shape the success or failure of independent restaurants that feature organic foods in metropolitan cities in the United States.

Meanwhile, the educational background of the restaurant owners had a statistically significant relationship with profits ($r = .359$, $p = .031$). Leadership traits such as honesty had a statistically significant relationship with profits ($r = -.404$, $p = .015$). Furthermore, the days the restaurants were opened for business to serve customers had a statistically significant relationship with profits ($r = .442$, $p = .007$).

The results of the correlation analysis in Table 1.6 above show that there was a statistically significant relationship between risk taking, which was used as a proxy for leadership traits, and the average cost associated with their operations ($r = -.349$, $p = .037$). This suggests that perhaps the risk-taking behavior or behavioral intentions of restaurant owners in the sample were only correlated ($p < .05$) with the average cost associated with their operations.

The results in the table above also show that there was statistically significant relationship between the risk-taking behavior and the number of customers served per week ($r = -.336$, $p = .045$). From this conclusion, one could deduce that the more the restaurant owners were willing to take risks, the larger the number of customers they serve, and perhaps the lower their average costs. Furthermore, there was a statistically significant relationship between the number of training programs enrolled into and the risk-taking behavior of restaurant owners ($r = .384$, $p = .021$).

Table 1.6 also demonstrates that there was a statistically significant relationship between the risk-taking behavior as a proxy for leadership traits of restaurant owners and their sense of responsibility ($r = .386$, $p = .020$). Readers should note, however, that in as much as these findings in no way allowed the researcher to accept or reject the stipulated null hypotheses, they shed an important light on the consequences of the risk-taking behaviors of owners of independent restaurants that feature organic foods in metropolitan cities in the United States.

The analysis also found that there was a statistically significant relationship between the risk-taking behavior of restaurants and honesty ($r = .368$, $p = .027$). Table 1.6 also shows that the relationship between leadership traits and life cycle was not statistically significant ($r = .229$, $p = -.205$).

Table 1.7
Regression Equation Predicting Classification (Results of Stepwise Regression; N = 36)

Variables	Coefficient	Standard Error	p-value
Intercept	-.951	.470	.006
Average cost	.872	.126	.000
Menu category	.190	.050	.001
Customers served	-.236	.080	.005

R-Square = .702
Adj. R. Square = .674
F statistic = 8.917
Sig F = .005

$p <.05^*$, $p <.01^{**}$

Results of the stepwise regression analysis are contained in Table 1.7. The results demonstrate the extent to which the value of the dependent variable classification of independent restaurants into Quick Service, Midscale, and Upscale could be predicated from the values of the independent variables, when some of these variables were controlled for. Thus, in this equation, the average cost associated with the sale of each meal (b = .872, p = .000) was a significant predictor of how participants in the survey described their restaurants in terms of one of the three categories defined above (Quick Service, Midscale, and Upscale).

The menu category of the restaurants was also a significant predictor of how the survey participants described their restaurants in terms of belonging to one of the three categories defined above. The regression equation for the menu category was (b = .190, p = .001).

On the other hand, customers served per week (b = -.238, p = .005) was not a significant predictor of how the survey participants described their restaurants in terms of belonging to one of the categories referred to above. The adjusted R^2 for the model in Table 1.7 was .702, or 70%, and a significant F = 8.917, p = .005.

Table 1.8

Regression Equation Predicting Days of Operation (Results of Stepwise Regression; N = 36)

Variables	Coefficient	Standard Error	p-value
Intercept	-.097	.1.200	.936
Average cost	1.125	.391	.007

R-Square =.196
Adj. R. Square = .173
F statistic = 8.298
Sig F = .007

p <.05*, p <.01**

Results of the stepwise regression analysis are contained in Table 1.8. In Table 1.8, the average cost (b = 1.125, p = .007) associated with the sale of each meal is shown to be the most significant predictor of how participants described the days of operation peer week of their independent restaurants. The adjusted R^2 was .173, or 17%, and a significant $F = 8.298$, $p = 007$. Consistent with the results of the correlation analysis reported above, this result allowed the researcher to reject the null hypothesis (H_0) and stipulate that there is partial support for the alternative hypothesis (H_{2a}) due to the relatively small sample size.

Table 1.9

Regression Equation Predicting Leadership Traits (Results of Stepwise Regression; N = 36)

Variables	Coefficient	Standard Error	p-value
Intercept	1.091	.671	.114
Average cost	-.079	.128	.541
Training	.103	.069	.149
Customers served	-.105	.067	.131
Responsibility	.344	.122	.008
Honesty	.168	.145	.186

R-Square = .654
Adj. R. Square = .333
F statistic = 4.495
Sig F = .004

p <.05* p <.01**

Table 1.9 presents results of the regression analysis. A simple multiple linear regression analysis was performed at the p-value ($p = .05$) because a more robust stepwise regression analysis at a much lower p-value ($p = .01$) could not be performed as it excluded all the independent variables. The results of this analytical approach show that average cost was not a significant predictor of risk-taking behavior used as a proxy for leadership traits ($b = -.079$, $p = .541$). These results rejected the stipulated null hypotheses. However, they shed an important light on the variables that are affected by average cost associated with the sale of each meal to customers.

Meanwhile, the number of training programs employees attended was also not a significant predictor of risk-taking behavior ($b = .103$, $p = .149$). The number of customers served per week was also not a significant predictor of risk-taking behavior of restaurant owners (b = -.105, p = .131). However, the sense of responsibility displayed as per their preference on the survey items exhibited by the restaurant owners was a significant predictor of risk-taking behavior (b = .344, p = .008). The honesty of restaurant owners as an independent variable was not a significant predictor of risk-taking behavior (b = .168, p = .256). The adjusted R^2 was .333, or 33%, and a significant F = 4.495, p = 004. These results in no way allowed the researcher to accept or reject the null hypotheses in an attempt to address the research questions.

Table 1.10

Regression Equation Predicting Profits (Results of Stepwise Regression; N = 36)

Variables	Coefficient	Standard Error	p-value
Intercept	126506.997	17436.756	.007
Days of operation	13565.662	.4726.274	.007

R-Square = .442
Adj. R. Square = .171
F statistic = 8.238
Sig F = .007

p <.05*, p <.01**

Table 1.10 above shows the results of the regression analysis to determine the predictors of profits. Days of operation (b = -.13565.662, p = .007) was the only significant predictor of the profits of the restaurants represented in the sample. The adjusted R^2 for the model in Table 1.10 was .171, or 17%, and a significant F = 8.238, p = .007. The current study showed that most respondents (66.7%; SD = .478) in the sample used social media to promote their products, whereas only 33.3% (SD = .478) of respondents used word of mouth. Figure 1.2 below presents a frequency diagram that depicted these results. However, it is worth noting that this study did not find any statistically significant relationship (p> .05) between the profits of independent restaurants in the sample and the form of advertisement the respondents used to promote their products.

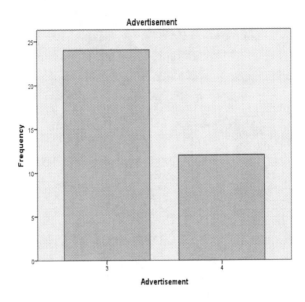

Figure 1.2. Advertisement by independent restaurant owners.

Figure 1.2 above shows that most respondents (66.7%; *SD* = .478) in the sample used social media to promote their products, whereas only 33.3% (*SD* = .478) of respondents used word of mouth. Figure 1.3 below presents a frequency diagram depicting these results. Correlation analysis was computed to determine the relationship between the variable, classification, and the various thoughts about organic foods among the respondents (*N* = 36).

The results found that there was no statistically significant relationship between classification and the various thoughts about organic foods among the respondents. Most of the respondents (61.1%) agreed they decided to go into the organic restaurant business because organic food is in high demand. Further, 30.6% of respondents agreed they decided to get into the organic restaurant business because organic food is much healthier than nonorganic food. Meanwhile, only 3% of participants agreed that organic food is easy or difficult to produce. Figure 1.3 below depicts the distribution of these responses.

Figure 1.3 demonstrates that most respondents (66.7%; *SD* = .478) in the sample used social media to promote their products, whereas only 33.3% (*SD* = .478) of respondents used word of mouth.

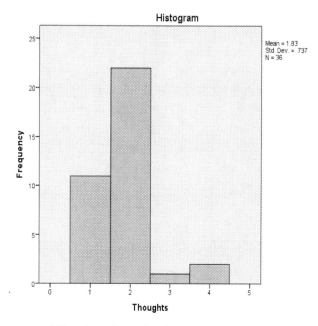

Figure 1.3. The thoughts of independent restaurant owners.

A one-way ANOVA was computed comparing the mean average cost of the three groups of restaurants identified in the sample (Quick Service, Midservice, and Upscale). A significant difference was found among the three categories of restaurants [$F(2, 33)$ = 15.37, $p < .05$]. Tukey's HSD test was used to determine the nature of the differences between the groups. Thus, this analysis revealed that the restaurants that chose less than $11.00 as their average cost per item on the menu scored lower (m = 1.38, SD = .518) than those that chose more than $12.00-$19.00 (m = 1.85, SD =.745). In addition, those that chose more than $12.00-$19.00 scored lower than those that chose more than $20.00 ($m$ = 3.00, SD = .828).

Tables 1.11 and 1.12 below attempted to encapsulate the essential research findings in terms of our attempt to address the two stipulated research questions and their corresponding null and alternative hypotheses.

Research Question One

To what extent do factors such as the average cost associated with the sale of each meal, profits and life cycle influence independent restaurants that feature organic foods in metropolitan areas in the United States?

Overall findings on Research Question One. In responding to Research Question One, we formulated and tested two null hypotheses. The results are reported in Table 1.11. Correlation analysis was primarily used to test the hypotheses. A stepwise regression analysis was also used. The findings showed that average cost associated with the sale of each organic meal was highly correlated with the number of days the restaurants were opened. Similarly, the stage the restaurants were at in their maturation process (life cycle) had no statistically significant relationship with the profits earned by the independent restaurants in the sample during the fiscal period of 2015.

Table 1.11

Results of Hypotheses Testing For Question One

Hypotheses	Testing Used	Results of Testing	Accept/Reject Hypotheses
H2$_o$: The average cost associated with the sale of each meal has no impact on the days of operation of independent restaurants featuring organic foods (RQ1).	**Correlation Analysis** **Regression Analysis (p<.01)**	r=.443, p=.007** (significant at p<.01) Average cost (b=1.125, p=.007) (R^2 =17%).	Reject Hypothesis
H$_{2a}$: The average cost associated with the sale of each meal has a significant impact on the days of operation of independent restaurants featuring organic foods (RQ1)	**Correlation Analysis** **Regression Analysis (p<.01)**	r=.443, p=.007** (significant at p<.01) Average cost (b=1.125, p=.007) (R^2 =17%).	Accept Hypothesis
H$_{4o}$: The life cycle of independent restaurants featuring organic foods has no impact on their profits (RQ1).	**Correlation Analysis** **Regression Analysis (p<.01)**	r=.282, p=.095 (not significant) Days of operation (b=13565.662, p=.007) (R^2=17%).	Accept Hypothesis

H$_{4a}$: The life cycle of independent restaurants featuring organic foods has a significant impact on their profits. (RQ1).	**Correlation Analysis** **Regression Analysis** **(p<.01)**	r=.282, p=.095 (not significant) Days of operation (b=13565.662, p=.007) (R^2=17%)	Reject Hypothesis

Research Question Two

To what extent do average cost associated with the sale of each meal and profits influence the classification of independent restaurants that feature organic foods in metropolitan cities in the United States into Quick Service, Midservice, and Upscale?

Overall findings on Research Question Two. In responding to Research Question Two, we formulated and tested two null hypotheses. The results are reported in Table 1.12. Correlation analysis was primarily used to test the hypotheses. A stepwise-regression analysis was also used. The findings showed that average cost associated with the sale of each organic meal was correlated with classification of the independent restaurants in the sample into the three categories of Quick Service, Midservice, and Upscale. Similarly, the profits earned by the independent restaurants in the sample in the 2015 fiscal period were also correlated with their classification. Thus, upon this basis, the null hypothesis was rejected and the alternative hypothesis was accepted.

Table 1.12

Results of Hypotheses Testing For Question Two

Hypotheses	Testing Used	Results of Testing	Accept/Reject Hypotheses
H₁ₒ: The average cost associated with the sale of each meal has no impact on the classification of independent restaurants featuring organic foods. (RQ2).	**Correlation Analysis** **Regression Analysis (p<.01)**	r=.663, p=.000** (significant at p<.01) Average cost (b=.872, p=.000). Menu Category (b=.190, p=.001). Customers served (b=-.236, p=.005). (significant at p<.01) (R^2=67%)	Reject Hypothesis
H₁ₐ: The average cost associated with the sale of each meal has an impact on the classification of independent restaurants featuring organic foods. (RQ2)	**Correlation Analysis** **Regression Analysis (p<.01)**	r=.663, p=.000** (significant at p<.01) Average cost (b=.872, p=.000). Menu Category (b=.190, p=.001). Customers served (b=-.236, p=.005). (significant at p<.01) (R^2=67%)	Accept Hypothesis
H₃ₒ: The profits from the operations of independent restaurants featuring organic foods has no relationship with their classification. (RQ2).	**Correlation Analysis** **Regression Analysis (p<.01)**	r=.387, p=.020* (significant at p<.05) Average cost (b=.872, p=.000). Menu category (b=.190, p=.001). Customers served (b=-.236, p=.080). (significant at p<.01).	Reject Hypothesis
H₃ₐ: The profits from the operations of independent restaurants featuring organic foods has a significant relationship with their classification (RQ2).	**Correlation Analysis** **Regression Analysis (p<.01)**	r=.387, p.020* (significant at p<.05) Average cost (b=.872, p=.000). Menu category (b=.190, p=.001). Customers served (b=-.236, p=.080). (significant at p<.01)	Accept Hypothesis

Summary and Conclusion

This chapter provided results of the data analysis and a restatement of the research purpose in an attempt to respond to the research question and hypotheses. Descriptive statistics were also presented on the dependent and independent variables. The research questions and hypotheses were also restated. In addition, the results of correlation analysis were presented in Tables 1.3, 1.4, 1.5, and 1.6.

The results of the stepwise regression analysis were presented in Tables 1.7 and 1.8. Meanwhile, the results of a simple regression analysis were presented in Table 1.9. Thus, Table 1.3 showed the effects of average cost, life cycle, number of days the restaurants were opened per week, and profits made from operations on restaurant classification. Other independent variables that were not statistically significant were excluded from the table.

Furthermore, Table 1.3 showed that the effects of the independent variables on restaurant classification, such as the average cost of an item on the menu, which ranged from less than $6.00 to more than $20.00, and how often the restaurants changed their menus and the number of customers served per week, were more statistically significant when other variables were controlled for in the stepwise regression model. The results of the one-way ANOVA were also reported in this chapter. In addition, Chapter Four discussed the results of hypotheses testing in the context of existing literature. Recommendations for future research endeavors predicated on these findings were also posited in Chapter Four. The results of hypotheses testing on the basis of the correlation and regression analyses were reported in Tables 1.11 and 1.12 above. The overall findings in response to the two research questions were also discussed.

Chapter Five
Summary and Conclusions

Introduction

This chapter will provide a discussion of the research findings presented in Chapter Four. In Chapter One, we presented the problem background to this study in terms of the underlying reasons that led to the selection of the research topic. The two underlying research questions were also provided in Chapter One. Similarly, the chapter provided the purpose and nature of this study. In addition, the statement of the problem was also provided. Next, Chapter One presented the significance of the study as well as the research hypotheses. It was posited that the central objective of this study was to provide some contributions to the survey research literature in terms of the factors that affect independent restaurants.

Chapter Two discussed findings reported in prior academic studies that undergirded this study. Chapter Three presented the methodological framework on which this study was built. The framework was one of a quantitative research approach. The chapter also presented a restatement of the research problem. In addition, the chapter further discussed the research design, including the characteristics and type of survey instrument adopted. The methodological assumptions that attempted to ensure validity of the research findings were also posited in Chapter Three. The chapter discussed the process of selection of the research participants as well as data analysis.

Chapter Four provided the results of data analysis. Descriptive statistics as well as inferential statistics were provided and analyzed in this chapter. The current chapter will discuss the research findings in the context of existing academic studies that have focused on the multiplicity of variables that ultimately influence the relative successes and failures of independent restaurants featuring organic foods. In addition, the current chapter will provide a restatement of the research problem.

Restatement of the Research Problem

One of the problems that invariably provided the rationale for this research is the current paucity of data on the organic food business. One is led to believe that there is an indication that organic foods are being purchased on a relatively large scale (see Budhwar, 2004), which is why there may be limited survey research investigating the pattern of demand in this sector. Consumers today are taking more care to know where their food comes from and what is in that food. However, the problem is that little research has been conducted to investigate the variables that affect the current pattern of demand for organic foods, let alone how independent restaurants are positioning themselves to furnish the need in this market (Budhwar, 2004).

Because of the aforementioned problem, gathering data on this subject was an uphill task (Budhwar, 2004). One should recognize the fact that those consumers who are health and nutrition conscious possess necessary awareness and knowledge of foods and labels. However, for those consumers who are not health conscious, labels may not have an effect when selecting a lower calorie item from the menu (Ellison, 2013). Because of these and other reasons, a study of this nature to fill in some of these gaps in scholarly and popular knowledge, information, and understanding could not be more relevant at this point in time. Empirical research studies may also be needed to address some of the questions associated with the factors that affect the successes and failures of independent organic restaurants, as there is a paucity of empirical and theoretical studies in this field.

Discussion

A review of prior studies has helped to determine the host of internal and external factors that influenced successes and failures among independent restaurants (Angelo et al., 2008; Goldman, 1993). We hope that the current study will add to these findings. In a more recent study by Parsa et al. (2014), an essential ingredient for the success of independent restaurants was posited. Citing another author, Parsa et al. defined success as follows: "Success in business is defined in terms of rate of return on sales, and age or longevity of the firm" (p. 2). Other studies, including one by Jennings and Beaver (as cited in Parsa et al., 2014), examined the "intangible goals of the small business owners in defining success" (p. 2). Success was also defined in this study as "the sustained satisfaction…and the attainment of certain pre-defined objectives which satisfy stakeholder aspirations" (Jennings & Beaver as cited in Parsa et al., 2014).

There are variables that also account for the failure of independent restaurants (Parsa et al., 2005). However, Parsa et al. (2005) suggested that there is no universal definition of restaurant failure (p. 305). Thus, it is suggested that studies that use a "narrow definition of failure such as bankruptcy" tend to have the lowest failure rate, while those that focus on a broad definition, such as change of ownership, tend to have the highest failure rate. Parsa et al. (2011) suggested that reasons for organizational failures in the restaurant sector could be based on three factors—restaurant location, affiliation, and size.

These are some of the factors the authors deemed as critical to understanding organizational failure from a population ecology perspective (Parsa et al., 2014, p. 360). Unlike the construct of rate of return on sales, as adopted by Parsa et al. (2014), the current dissertation used profits and average cost among other variables to rank independent restaurants into three categories. This approach to gauging the success of the restaurants in the sample was used because the researcher could not gain access to information on rates of return. Thus, profits, for example, is used in this study as one of the many factors that define success. The three categories identified in the sample were: Quick Service, Midservice, and Upscale restaurants.

Descriptive statistics showed that the profits for the three categories of the independent organic restaurants in the sample for the year 2015 ranged from $80,000 for those categorized in the Quick Service category, more than $80,000 but less than $300,000 for those categorized as Midservice, and $300,000 for those categorized as Upscale. The researcher argues that while prior studies referred to independent restaurants broadly (Angelo et al., 2008; Parsa et al., 2014; Parsa et al., 2015; Rupali et al., 2015), the definition of success presented in these studies could also be applied to independent restaurants that feature organic foods.

The hypothesized role that profits played in the classification of the more successful organic restaurants was taken note of in this study. Hence, the results of correlation analyses showed that there was a statistically significant relationship between profits and the classification of the restaurants. However, this finding was not confirmed by the results of the regression analyses. Thus, regression analysis conducted to determine the predictors of classification of Quick Service, Midservice, and Upscale showed that three variables were predictors of the classification of independent restaurants into these categories: average cost, menu category, and number of customers served per week at each of the independent restaurants in the sample.

As readers would note, profits is nowhere included among these variables. In fact, further empirical analysis was conducted to determine how the three categories of restaurants in the sample varied on their average cost per item on the menu (Cronk, 2008). The first null hypothesis (H_0) in this study posited that the average cost associated with the sale of each item on the menu had no impact on the classification of independent restaurants featuring organic foods. The finding showed that average cost is significantly correlated ($p < .01$) with the classification of the independent restaurants ($N = 36$) sampled in this study. We thus hypothesize that the three categories of restaurants were associated with the average cost of services rendered at these restaurants. We further conclude that the mean average cost per item on the menu differed among the three categories of restaurants as confirmed by the results of the one-way ANOVA rendered in the previous chapter.

On the basis of this conclusion, we suggest that there is no support for the first null hypothesis and therefore partial support for the first alternative hypothesis (H_{01}). As has been indicated above, there are other factors that also account for successes and failures among independent restaurants. Thus, Angelo et al. (2008) have enumerated several characteristics that also account for successful and failed restaurant owners (p. 373). These included the fact that restaurant owners in their sample were perceived as being highly motivated, positively charged, and emotionally stable.

Other critical success factors named in this article included strategic choices by restaurant owners, knowledge of competitive forces, productive relevance, marketing abilities, public relations, advertising, and firm size

(Angelo et al., 208, p. 367). Other factors listed included organizational culture, financial management and profitability, internal controls, efficiency, and service levels. Parsa et al. (2012) found that one of the factors that could account for increased sales in Upscale and Quick Service restaurants is if more resources are focused on attributes that are appropriate for that segment.

The current study also attempted to examine other factors that impinged upon respondents' perception of their risk-taking behavior. Thus, the results of the correlation analysis showed that there was statistically significant relationship between risk taking—which was used as a proxy for leadership traits—and the average cost associated with their operations. This result led the researchers to postulate that the risk-taking behavior or behavioral intentions of restaurant owners were correlated with the average cost associated with their operations. The willingness to take risk by owners also seemed to be a factor in attracting more customers.

From this conclusion, one could deduce that the more the restaurant owners were willing to take risks, the larger the number of customers they served, and perhaps the lower their average costs. Furthermore, there was a statistically significant relationship between the number of training programs employees were encouraged to enroll into by the restaurant owners and the risk-taking behavior of restaurant owners. Leadership traits or the risk-taking behavior of restaurant owners were also correlated with the owners' sense of personal responsibility. The results showed that there was a statistically significant relationship between the risk-taking behavior as a proxy for leadership traits of restaurant owners and their sense of personal responsibility. The analysis also found that there was statistically significant relationship between the risk-taking behavior of restaurants and honesty. Leadership traits or the risk-taking behavior of restaurant owners were correlated with the life cycle of the restaurants in the sample. The results reflected that the relationship between leadership traits and life cycle was not statistically significant.

The idea expressed by respondents that organic foods are in high demand has been confirmed by other empirical studies (Bernstein et al., 2008; Dimitri & Oberholtzer, 2009). Dimitri and Oberholtzer (2009) suggested that a broader range of consumers have been buying more varieties of organic foods. The authors also noted that organic handlers, who often purchase products from farmers with the intention of supplying them to retailers, sell more organic products to conventional retailers and club stores than ever before.

DiPietro and Gregory (2012) reported that upscale restaurant customers believed they are knowledgeable about green restaurant practices, environmental record, and recycling in restaurants. The authors also reported this cohort of consumers believed that restaurants should use local products when they can. Verdurme et al. (2002) recognized the growing demand for organic foods:

> Consumers have become increasingly concerned about health and its link with food. Moreover, environmental awareness is growing rapidly. Consequently, some consumers resort to organic agriculture, which is perceived as cleaner and healthier food. It is reflected by the upward demand for organic food products. (p. 610)

Sharma, Strohbehn, Radhakrishna, and Ortiz (2009) conducted a study to assess process and production costs incurred using locally produced foods versus food products sourced through national suppliers. This study concluded that there was no statistically significant difference in production efficiencies by scale, establishment effects, and preparation time of menu items using local versus nonlocal ingredients. The current study found that the average cost associated with the sale of each meal had a statistically significant relationship with the days of operation of the restaurants featuring organic foods.

While the current study considered the effects of size by associating Upscale restaurants that feature organic foods with those that benefited more from the economies of scale, it did not examine establishment effects (DiPietro & Gregory, 2012) or other factors that contribute to lower costs of production. Results of regression analysis tended to reinforce the correlation results, where the average cost associated with the sale of each meal was found to be a significant predictor of the days of operation of the restaurants.

We would expand on the point made above by proposing that perhaps the following finding—the more days the restaurants were opened for service, the less their average costs associated with the sale of each meal were—was a result of the economic phenomenon of economies of scale. On the basis of this discussion, one would conclude that the second null hypothesis (H_0) was not supported, while the alternative hypothesis (H_{02}) was partially supported.

As was indicated in Chapter One, one of the major challenges of this study was that fact that we could not obtain information on profits for more than one year from respondents. However, it is worth reemphasizing that profits are not the only indicator that one could use to judge the health of an independent business, even those that feature organic foods. We suggest that other processes are at work that should also be captured in analyses. Correlation analysis was conducted to test the third null hypothesis (H_0).

The results showed that profits had a significant relationship with the classification of the restaurants into three categories as already discussed in this chapter. The results showed that there was a significant relationship between profits and classification. On the basis of this result, we posit that the third null hypothesis was not supported. Thus, the alternative hypothesis (H_{03}) was supported. The fourth null hypothesis examined the impact of the life cycle (introduction, growing, maturity, and decline) of independent restaurants featuring organic foods on organizational profits.

The results of correlation analysis found that the life cycle of the restaurants as reported by respondents had no significant impact on profits. Meanwhile, a stepwise regression analysis was performed to determine the most significant predictors of profits. The results showed that only the days of operation of the restaurants were a significant predictor of profits. Hence, the life cycle of the restaurants together with other independent variables were not significant predictors. On the basis of these findings, the fourth null hypothesis (H_0) was not supported. Thus, the fourth alternative hypothesis (H_{04}) was partially supported.

Implications for Professional Practice and Organizational Leadership

Among many efforts, we also examined implications of the research findings for professional practice. It is worth noting that as with many studies of its kind, the current study possesses implications for professional practice in terms of how leadership decisions impact the structuring of an organizational climate that embraces success. Several studies have emphasized the critical ingredients that instigate organizational success in the independent segment of the restaurant industry (Angelo et al., 2008; Bayou & Bennett, 1992; Bertsimas & Shioda, 2003; Parsa, 2005). We note that these critical ingredients are also imperative for organic foods in independent restaurants.

Angelo et al. (2008) discussed some of the critical factors that affect the failure rate of independent restaurants. The authors developed a restaurant viability model that identified family life cycle, organizational life cycle, and internal and external processes as determinants of restaurant viability. These observations are in line with those made by Parsa et al. (2005) who argued that past research on restaurant failures focused mainly on quantitative factors, ignoring other important qualitative factors (p. 369).

This perspective tended to be buttressed by authors like Keasey and Watson (as cited in Parsa et al., 2005, p. 369) who have suggested that traditional financial models may not be appropriate for making a comprehensive assessment of the viability of new and small ventures. These assumptions lead to one important fact: Leadership is a critically important variable in terms of the underlying factors that account for organizational success. Cichy et al. (1992) enumerated four areas of competencies that leaders should possess: attention through vision, meaning through communication, trust through positioning, and the development of self through positive self-regard (p. 48). Leaders are expected to have an ability to create a sense of outcome through which others are drawn in and become similarly committed (Cichy et al., 1992, p. 48).

Leaders are also able to communicate their sense of vision with clarity and purpose (Cichy et al., 1992, p. 48). Further, the authors also noted that leaders should be required to consistently demonstrate and earn trust through their reliability, predictability, and accountability (Cichy et al., 1992, p. 48). Similarly, the authors noted that inconsistency breeds misunderstanding and distrust, which are obstacles that are not easily overcome (Cichy et al., 1992, p. 48). Effective leaders are also perceived as ones who know their strengths and consistently work to enhance them (Cichy et al., 1992, p. 48). Leaders are also perceived as those who recognize their shortcomings and seek to compensate for them (Cichy et al., 1992, p.

48). It is suggested that the capacity to improve upon their skills is what distinguishes "leaders" from "followers" (Cichy et al., 1992, p. 48)

Gill et al. (2011) suggested that the importance of retaining staff cannot be ignored. Indeed, they also posited that transformational leadership has a direct impact on the empowerment of employees and their willingness to quit. These authors examined the effects of many different factors on employee intention to quit, which in turn leads to high employee turnover. The authors further posited that high employee turnover is not in the favor of service organizations like independent restaurants because it has a direct impact on high hiring and training costs. These perspectives line up with some of the findings of the current research. Thus, as discussed above, the willingness of restaurant owners to exhibit responsibility and honesty and to encourage further training for their employees could be perceived as some of the effective leadership strategies required for the success of their restaurants.

Another important aspect of transformational and effective leadership is the organizational culture that leaders, be they owners of independent or chain restaurants, can help create in the organization. Clement (1994) suggested that the researcher should focus on an organization's culture in order to emphasize organizational practices rather than values. This idea was borrowed from studies conducted by Hofstede et al. (1990) who extensively studied organizational culture and its dimensions. Writing about how an organizational culture encourages innovation and change, Boisnier and Chatman (2002) defined the concept of organizational culture as follows:

> A good way to grasp the concept of company culture is to think of a firm as a mini-civilization. All civilizations have a group of animating beliefs and values that gives meaning, purpose, and direction. These beliefs constitute culture. The United States, for example, is centered on the beliefs and values found in the Declaration of Independence and our Constitution. If you reduce those beliefs down to their essence, you might say that our national animating principles are "equality before the law," "life, liberty and the pursuit of happiness," among others. (pp. 121-122)

Boisnier and Chatman (2002) further suggested that culture is an essential ingredient for organizational success because it offers a sense of permanence, direction, and marketplace identity, and also helps us find our natural allies (pp. 123-134). Roxborough (2000) suggested that organizational culture is critically important to fostering the debates necessary for successful innovation within the organization. Kaarst et al. (2004) researched the organizational cultures of libraries and concluded that organizational culture is a strategic resource that must be harnessed. Organizational culture can also be a basis for legitimacy-seeking, as suggested by institutional theory (Dickson et al., 2004).

Goldman (1993) conducted research on the concept selection for independent restaurants and concluded that for independent restaurants to thrive, they must have a clear-cut identity and a defined concept that caters to a specific group. Ogbeide and Harrington (2011) conducted research on management in the food service industry and concluded that larger organizational structures require higher levels of involvement by middle and lower management levels to successfully make use of strategic processes.

Ogbeide and Harrington (2011) further suggested that food service firms in their study adopt a participative management style similar to that of larger or smaller food service firms. In a study of quick service restaurants, DiPietro and Strate (2006) found that the positive perception held by managers with respect to older workers does not translate into a stated desire to actually hire a larger percentage of older workers to staff the restaurants. Cumberland and Herd (2011) viewed the culture of the organization as a tool for determining which interventions may be appropriate during a merger, acquisition, or divestiture. The authors noted the importance of the study of organizational culture in small franchise restaurants and other restaurant types as well.

Recommendations for Future Research

We suggest that future studies should focus on obtaining time series data on costs and profits that reflect a longer time horizon, perhaps five years or more. It is doubtless that such data might yield more accurate results. We further suggest that future research should also focus not just on independent restaurants that feature organic foods in general, but also on independent ethnic restaurants that feature organic foods in metropolitan cities in the United States. This recommendation follows from the realization informed by the available data that there are many ethnic independent restaurants that are involved in the organic food business. However, empirical studies on this topic are difficult to come by.

In fact, and perhaps as already indicated, one should note that empirical studies on independent organic restaurants are also few and far between. We also call for more comparative research that focuses on making cross-country comparisons. The aim of such efforts would be to examine both managers' and customers' perceptions about issues of sustainability, concerns about the environment, healthy foods, and animal rights activities around the world and how these affect menu choices.

Summary and Conclusion

This chapter presented a summary of previous chapters. The chapter also discussed the results of the data analysis in an attempt to explain some of the factors that affect independent restaurants that feature organic foods in the United States. Thus, the current chapter discussed the research findings in the context of existing empirical studies. The chapter also presented some of the factors that account for the failure of restaurants.

Further, the discussion in this chapter urged scholars to go beyond the construct of rate of return to focus on other quantitative and qualitative factors that account for success in independent restaurants. This chapter put forth the notion that studies about the factors that undergird the success and failures of independent restaurants should include quantitative and qualitative variables that transcend financial modeling. The chapter presented the results of hypotheses testing, which was performed using correlation and regression analyses.

It was also indicated that a one-way ANOVA was computed comparing the mean average cost of the three groups of restaurants in the sample. The study showed that most of the respondents in the sample used social media to promote their products. This study considered the effects of size, but not establishment effects or other factors that lower the cost of production of independent restaurants that feature organic foods. The chapter discussed implications of the research findings for professional practice and organizational leadership.

The chapter made a case for further studies focusing on ethnic independent restaurants that are involved in the organic food business. We also called for more comparative research programs that focus on making cross-country comparisons. It is suggested that the aim of such efforts would be to examine the impact of contemporary political and social issues on how agents make their menu choices. We also emphasized the fact that future studies should focus on how the demand for organic foods influences the strategic and managerial choices of restaurant owners.

Bibliography

Aertsens, J., Mondelaers, K., Verbeke, W., Buysse, J., & Guido, V. H. (2011). The influence of subjective and objective knowledge on attitude, motivations and consumption of organic food. *British Food Journal, 113*(11), 1353-1378.

Agarwal, R., & Dahm, M. J. (2015). Success factors in independent ethnic restaurants. *Journal of Foodservice Business Research, 18*(1), 20-33.

Bagby, R. M., Taylor, G. J., & Parker, J. D. A. (1992). *Reliability and validity of the 20-item revised Toronto Alexithymia Scale.* Paper presented at the meeting of the American Psychosomatic Society, New York.

Beaver, G., & Jennings, P. (2000). Editorial overview: Small business, entrepreneurship and enterprise development. *Strategic Change, 9*(7), 397.

Boisnier, A., & Chatman, J. (2002). The role of subcultures in agile organizations.

Budhwar, K. (2005). Understanding the success factors for independent restaurants in the Delhi/Gurgoan region: An analysis of the gap between management perceptions and customer expectations. *Journal of Services Research, 4*(2), 7-30, 32-36, 44.

Camillo, A. A., Connolly, D. J., & Kim, W. G. (2008). Success and failure in Northern California: Critical success factors for independent restaurants. *Cornell Hospitality Quarterly, 49*(4), 364-380.

Carvalho, D. R., & Rodrigues Silva, M. A. (2014). Eating-out and experiential consumption: A typology of experience providers. *British Food Journal, 116*(1), 91-103.

Cichy, R. F., Sciarini, M. P., & Patton, M. E. (1992). Food-service leadership: Could Attila run a restaurant?. *The Cornell Hotel and Restaurant Administration Quarterly, 33*(1), 47-55.

Clement, R. W. (1994). Culture, leadership, and power: The keys to organizational change. *Business Horizons, 37*(1), 33-39.

Cronk, B. C. (2008). *How to use SPSS: A step-by-step guide to analysis and interpretation* (5ᵗʰ ed.). Pyrczak Publishing.

Cumberland, D., & Herd, A. (2011). Organizational culture: Validating a five windows qualitative cultural assessment tool with a small franchise restaurant case study. *Organization Development Journal, 29*(4), 9.

Dickson, M. W., BeShears, R. S., & Gupta, V. (2004). The impact of societal culture and industry on organizational culture: Theoretical explanations. *Culture, Leadership, and Organizations: The GLOBE Study, 62*, 4-93.

Dimitri, C., & Dettmann, R. L. (2012). Organic food consumers: What do we really know about them? *British Food Journal, 114*(8), 1157-1183.

Dimitri, C., & Greene, C. (2002). Recent growth patterns in the U.S. organic foods market. *Agriculture Information Bulletin, 777.* Washington, DC: Department of Agriculture, Economic Research Service.

DiPietro, R. B., & Strate, M. L. (2006). 11. Management perceptions of older employees in America's restaurant industry. In *Older workers, new directions: Employment and development in an aging labor market.* Miami, FL: Center for Labor Research and Studies, Florida International University.

Dziadkowiec, J., & Rood, A. S. (2015). Casual-dining restaurant preferences: A cross- cultural comparison. *Journal of Foodservice Business Research, 18*(1), 73-91.

Ellison, B., Lusk, J. L., & Davis, D. (2013). Looking at the label and beyond: The effects of calorie labels, health consciousness, and demographics on caloric intake in restaurants. *International Journal of Behavioral Nutrition and Physical Activity, 10*, 21.

Field, A. (2009). *Discovering statistics using SPSS* (3ʳᵈ ed.). Los Angeles: Sage.

Food and Drug Administration. (2016). About FDA. Retrieved from: http://www.fda.gov/NewsEvents/ProductsApprovals/

Forks Over Knives. (2011). Retrieved from http://www.forksoverknives. com/about-us/

Gill, A., Fitzgerald, S., Bhutani, S., Mand, H., & Sharma, S. (2011). The relationship between transformational leadership and employee desire for empowerment. *International Journal of Contemporary Hospitality Management, 22*(2), 263-273.

Goldman, K. (1993). Concept selection for independent restaurants. *Cornell Hotel and Restaurant Administration Quarterly, 34*(6), 59-72.

Gregory, C., Rahkovsky, I., & Anekwe, T., (2014). Calorie labeling on restaurant menus: Who's likely to use it? Retrieved from http://www.ers.usda.gov/amber-waves/2014-september/calorie-labeling-on- restaurant/

Halse, C., & Honey, A. (2005). Unraveling Ethics: Illuminating the Moral Dilemmas of Research Ethics. *Signs: Journal Of Women In Culture & Society, 30*(4), 2141-2162.

Inwood, S. (2004). *Assessing opportunities for organic and sustainably grown local foods for restaurant and retail food store distribution in Ohio* (Doctoral dissertation). Retrieved from https://etd.ohiolink.edu/

Inwood, S. M., Sharp, J. S., Moore, R. H., & Stinner, D. H. (2009). Restaurants, chefs and local foods: Insights drawn from application of a diffusion of innovation framework. *Agriculture and Human Values, 26*(3), 177-191. Retrieved from: http://dx.doi.org/10.1007/s10460-008-9165-6

Jinghan, L., Zepeda, L., & Gould, B. W. (2007). The demand for organic food in the U.S.: An empirical assessment. *Journal Of Food Distribution Research, 38*(3), 54-69.

Kaarst-Brown, M. L., Nicholson, S., Von Dran, G. M., & Stanton, J. M. (2004). *Organizational cultures of libraries as a strategic resource.*

Kareklas, I., Carlson, J. R., & Muehling, D. D. (2014). "I eat organic for my benefit and yours": Egoistic and altruistic considerations for purchasing organic food and their implications for advertising strategists. *Journal of Advertising, 43*(1), 18-32.

Kotler, B., Bowen, I., & Makens. (1996). 1999 Marketing for hospitality and tourism.

Kriwy, P., & Mecking, R. (2012). Health and environmental consciousness, costs of behavior, and the purchase of organic food. *International Journal Of Consumer Studies, 36*(1), 30-37.

Mathe, K. (2012). Food safety, labor costs, and the effects on quick service restaurant revenues. *Journal of Foodservice Business Research, 15*(4), 398-410.

Merriam, S. B. A. (2002). *Qualitative research in practice: Examples for discussion and analysis* (1st ed.). San Francisco, CA: Jossey-Bass

Muller, C. C., & Woods, R. H. (1994). An expanded restaurant typology. *Cornell Hotel and Restaurant Administration Quarterly, 35*(3), 27.

Ogbeide, G. C. A., & Harrington, R. J. (2011). The relationship among participative management style, strategy implementation success, and financial performance in the foodservice industry. *International Journal of Contemporary Hospitality Management, 23*(6), 719-738.

Organic Trade Association (2016). Improvonia joins the organic trade association to improve access to organic products. Retrieved on November 4, 2016 from https://www.ota.com/news/industry-news/17811.

Organic Trade Association. (2016). Market analysis 2016. Retrieved from https://www.ota.com/resources/market-analysis

Parsa, H. G, Self, J., Gregory, A., & Dutta, K. (2012). Consumer behavior In restaurants: Assessing the importance of restaurant attributes in consumer patronage and willingness to pay. *Journal Of Services Research, 4*(2).

Parsa, H. G., Self, J., Sydnor-Busso, S., & Yoon, H. J. (2011). Why restaurants fail? Part II - The impact of affiliation, location, and size on restaurant failures: Results from a survival analysis. *Journal of Foodservice Business Research, 14*(4), 360- 379.

Parsa, H. G., Self, J. T., Njite, D., & King, T. (2005). Why restaurants fail. *Cornell Hotel and Restaurant Administration Quarterly, 46*(3), 304-322.

Parsa, H. G., van der Rest, J. P., Smith, S. R., Parsa, R. A., & Bujisic, M. (2015). Why restaurants fail? Part IV: The relationship between restaurant failures and demographic factors. *Cornell Hospitality Quarterly, 56*(1), 80-90.

Patton, L. (2015). Whole Foods, Walmart and Costco steal growth in organic groceries. *Bloomsberg Buisness Week*. Retrieved on November 4, 2008 from http://www.bloomberg.com/news/articles/2015-05-14/whole-foods-walmart-costco-steal-growth-in-organic-groceries

Poulston, J., & Yiu, A. Y. K. (2011). Profit or principles: Why do restaurants serve organic food? *International Journal of Hospitality Management, 30*(1), 184-191.

Roseman, M. G. (2006). Changing times: Consumers choice of ethnic foods when eating at restaurants. *Journal of Hospitality & Leisure Marketing, 14*(4), 5-32.

Roxborough, I. (2000, June). Organizational innovation: Lessons from military organizations. *Sociological Forum, 15*(2), 367-372.

Sharma, A., Strohbehn, C., Radhakrishna, R. B., & Ortiz, A. (2012). Economic viability of selling locally grown produce to local restaurants. *Journal of Agriculture, Food Systems, and Community Development, 3*(1), 181-198.

Small Business Administration. (2012). Do economic or industry factors affect business survival? Retrieved from http://www.sba.gov/sites/default/files/Business-Survival.pdf

USDA. (2009). U.S. market growth outpaces domestic supply. Retrieved October 29, 2016 from http://www.ers.usda.gov/media/452875/eib55b_1_.pdf

USDA. (2014). National Organic Program. Retrieved on October 29, 2016 from http://www.ams.usda.gov/AMSv1.0/ams.fetchTemplate Data.do?

USDA. (2014). Organic market overview. Retrieved on October 29, 2016 from http://www.ers.usda.gov/topics/natural-resources-environment/organic- agriculture/organic-market-overview.aspx

Verbeke, (2000). A revision of Hofstede et al.'s (1990) organizational practices scale. *Journal Of Organizational Behavior, 21*(5), 587.

Watson, P., Morgan, M., & Hemmington, N. (2008). Online communities and the sharing of extraordinary restaurant experiences. *Journal of Foodservice, 19*(6), 289.

Wells, J. (2013). Organic produce surges, but challenges remain. *SN: Supermarket News, 61*(38/39), 30.

Appendix 1
Letter of Permission

March 2016

Dear Chicago Organic Restaurant Participant,

You are cordially invited to participate in this research study, which is conducted by doctoral student Nina Moore. This study is a requirement for completing a doctorate degree in Business Administration at Argosy University/Chicago. **The purpose of this study is to determine the successes and challenges an Independent restaurant will encounter while featuring organic foods.**

Should you participate in this research, you will be asked to answer a survey consisting of 40 general information survey questionnaire. This survey will consist of questions regarding your business, business practice and philosophy and information on your customers based on your opinion.

The survey should not take more than 30 minutes to complete. You may refuse to participate entirely, or choose to stop your participation at any point during the research, without fear of penalty or negative consequences of any kind. The information/data you provide for this research will be anonymous, and all the raw data will be kept in a secure file by the researcher. There will be no personal benefit for participation in this research.

Results of the research will be reported as aggregate summary data only, and no individually identifiable information will be presented. There will be no direct or immediate personal benefits from your participation in this research. Your participation in this research is strictly voluntary and all information given will be anonymous.

If you agree to participate and take part of this study, you will be presented with a consent form, which will explain the terms and conditions to participate, after which you will be given the opportunity to decide whether you wish to participate or not to participate in this study.

It would be much appreciated if you would complete the survey ASAP so as the data can be collected and the research can begin immediately.

Thank you very much in advance for your anticipated cooperation.

Doctoral Candidate
Nina Moore
ninammoore@mail.com
Argosy University/Chicago Campus

Appendix 2
Consent Form

ARGOSY UNIVERSITY-CHICAGO RESEARCH PARTICIPANT INFORMATION AND CONSENT FORM

TITLE OF STUDY: Successes and Challenges in Independent Restaurants Featuring Organic Food.

INTRODUCTION: I have been asked to participate in a dissertation research being conducted by researcher Nina Moore. The study is in partial fulfillment of a Doctorate Degree in Business Administration (DBA). The research study is attempting to discover details about the demand and challenges of organic food on the menu of Independent restaurants. *A sample of 100 Independent restaurant owners' and chefs will be required for the completion of this research.*

PURPOSE OF THE STUDY: The purpose of this study is to determine the success and challenges organic food featured in independent restaurants and three concept restaurants: quick service, mid-scale and up-scale.

The main research question of this study has been formulated as follows:

Are there successes and challenges by independent restaurants that feature organic local foods on its menu?

STUDY PROCEDURES: If I agree to participate in this study, my participation will consist of completing a survey. Once I have read this consent form I will acknowledge my acceptance to give my consent to the conditions of the survey. Completion of the survey should take approximately 60 minutes.

I can obtain a copy of the results in the aggregate by writing to the researcher of this study by contacting them at:

Nina Moore
3252 North Hamlin Ave.
Chicago, Illinois 60618
(773) 580-9175
ninammoore@mail.com and her Dissertation Chairman at:

Instrument

QUESTIONNAIRE ABOUT A STUDY ON INDEPENDENT
RESTAURANTS FEATURING ORGANIC FOOD

*The survey questions together with the relevant keys are provided
below: *

A. General Information

A-1. What is your zip code for your business?

A-2. Gender
- ☐ 1. Male   (1)
- ☐ 2. Female   (2)

A-3. What is your age? _____
- ☐ 1. 21-30   (1)
- ☐ 2. 31-40   (2)
- ☐ 3. 41-50   (3)
- ☐ 4. 51 +   (4)
- ☐ 5. Prefer not to disclose. (5)

A-4. What types of traits would you consider yourself to have as of today?

Use the following scale for response options:

1=Excellent   (5)
2=Good   (4)
3=Average   (3)
4=Fair   (2)
5=Poor   (1)

		1	2	3	4	5
1.	Leadership	☐	☐	☐	☐	☐
2.	Responsible	☐	☐	☐	☐	☐
3.	Values	☐	☐	☐	☐	☐
4.	Knowledge	☐	☐	☐	☐	☐
5.	Experience	☐	☐	☐	☐	☐
6.	Focus	☐	☐	☐	☐	☐
7.	Risk Taker	☐	☐	☐	☐	☐
8.	Business savvy	☐	☐	☐	☐	☐
9.	Lucky	☐	☐	☐	☐	☐
10.	Balance	☐	☐	☐	☐	☐
11.	Audacious	☐	☐	☐	☐	☐
12.	Vision	☐	☐	☐	☐	☐
13.	Caring	☐	☐	☐	☐	☐
14.	Honest	☐	☐	☐	☐	☐

B. Business (Factors)

B-1. Is this your first business you ever owned and operated? If not, how many years have your business has been in operation (in total)? _____.

  ☐ 1. 1-3 years   (1)
  ☐ 2. 4-6 years   (2)
  ☐ 3. 7-9 years   (3)

☐ 4. 10- 20 years   (4)

☐ 5. 21 + years   (5)

a. If so, were any of your other businesses in the food industry?

☐ 1. Yes   (1)

☐ 2. No   (2)

B-2. Where is your location?

☐ 1. Within a strip mall   (1)

☐ 2. Standalone   (2)

☐ 3. Next to competition   (3)

☐ 4. Busy corner / intersection   (4)

B-3. What is the classification of your Independent Restaurant?

☐ 1. Quick service (Perceived as fast-food / take out)   (1)

☐ 2. Mid-Scale (Clearly not QS or upscale no reservations   (2) and not required to sell alcohol)

☐ 3. Up-Scale (Not perceived as fast food/takeout   (3) reservations, credit cards accepted alcohol served)

B-4. What is the average cost of an item on the menu?

☐ 1. Less than $6.00   (1)

☐ 2. Less than $11.00   (2)

☐ 3. More than $15.00   (3)

☐ 4. More than $20.00   (4)

B-5. What types of meals are services?

☐ 1. Breakfast   (1)

☐ 2. Lunch   (2)

☐ 3. Dinner   (3)

☐ 4. Snack   (4)

B-6. Is any of the food on the menu?

□ 1. Organic   (1)

□ 2. Local   (2)

□ 3. Both   (3)

□ 4. None   (4)

B-7. How many items on your menu are organic? (This includes single ingredients).

□ 1. Couple   (1)

□ 2. Some   (2)

□ 3. Most   (3)

□ 4. All   (4)

□ 5. None   (5)

B-8. How many items on your menu are local?

□ 1. All of the ingredients   (1)

□ 2. Some of the ingredients   (2)

B-9. How often do you change your menu?

□ 1. Every day   (1)

□ 2. Every week   (2)

□ 3. Seasonally   (3)

□ 4. Never   (4)

B-10. Is there a difference between Organic and Local products?

□ 1. Yes   (1)

□ 2. No   (2)

B-11. If organic, must it require an approval from USDA?

□ 1. Yes   (1)

□ 2. No   (2)

B-12. If local, what is the range of local?

☐ 1. Less than 5 miles   (1)

☐ 2. Less than 10 miles   (2)

☐ 3. Less than 15 miles   (3)

☐ 4. Less than 20 miles   (4)

☐ 5. Not applicable   (5)

B-13. Do you find it difficult to obtain organic food?

☐ 1. Yes   (1)

☐ 2. No   (2)

B-14. What are your thoughts on Organic food?

☐ 1. Healthier product   (1)

☐ 2. In high demand   (2)

☐ 3. Easy to produce   (3)

☐ 4. Difficult to produce   (4)

B-15. How many menu categories do you have?

☐ 1. Beverage   (1)

☐ 2. Appetizer   (2)

☐ 3. Main dish   (3)

☐ 4. Sides   (4)

☐ 5. Dessert   (5)

☐ 6. All of the above   (6)

B-16. What method of advertisement do you use for your restaurant?

☐ 1. Local newspaper   (1)

☐ 2. T.V. / Radio   (2)

☐ 3. Social Media   (3)

☐ 4. Word of Mouth   (4)

☐ 5. Not applicable   (5)

C. Business (Operations)

C-1. How many customers do to serve in:

a. a week _____?

☐ 1. 100-300   (1)

☐ 2. 301-500   (2)

☐ 3. 501-700   (3)

☐ 4. 701-1,000   (4)

☐ 5. 1,001 +   (5)

b. a year _____?

☐ 1. 1,000 -3,000   (1)

☐ 2. 3,001-5,000   (2)

☐ 3. 5,001-7,000   (3)

☐ 4. 7,001-10,000   (4)

☐ 5. 10,001 +   (5)

C-2. How many days are you open per week?

☐ 1. 7 days a week   (1)

☐ 2. 5 days a week   (2)

☐ 3. Weekends Only   (3)

☐ 4. Weekdays Only   (4)

☐ 5. I make my own schedule due to the season or other factor. (5)

Explain _____.

C-3. How many seats are available for sit- in_____?

☐ 1. Less than 10   (1)

☐ 2. 11-20   (2)

☐ 3. 21-30   (3)

☐ 4. 31+   (4)

C-4. How many employees do you employ on a daily basis?

☐ 1. Just me.   (1)

☐ 2. 2-5   (2)

☐ 3. 6-8   (3)

☐ 4. 9 +   (4)

C-5. How many times does your employees have training?

☐ 1. Once a week   (1)

☐ 2. Once a month   (2)

☐ 3. Quarterly   (3)

☐ 4. Annually   (4)

C-6. Do you have a high employee turn over rate?

☐ 1. Yes   (1)

☐ 2. No   (2)

C-7. Where would you say your business is at in its life cycle?

☐ 1. Introduction   (1)

☐ 2. Growing   (2)

☐ 3. Maturity   (3)

☐ 4. Decline   (4)

C-8. How did you finance your business?

☐ 1. 100%   (1)

☐ 2. 75%   (2)

☐ 3. 50%   (3)

☐ 4. 25%   (4)

☐ 5. 0%   (5)

C-9. Did someone else conduct any studies done before you opened your business?

☐ 1. Yes   (1)

☐ 2. No   (2)

C-10. What types of traits would you consider your business operations to have as of today?

Use the following scale for response options:

1=Excellent   (5)   3=Average   (3)   5=Poor   (1)

2=Good   (4)   4=Fair   (2)

		1	2	3	4	5
1.	Business Plan	☐	☐	☐	☐	☐
2.	Marketing Plan	☐	☐	☐	☐	☐
3.	Business Strategy	☐	☐	☐	☐	☐
4.	Customer relation/ communication	☐	☐	☐	☐	☐
5.	Experience	☐	☐	☐	☐	☐
6.	Focus	☐	☐	☐	☐	☐

D. Other Business Factors

D-1. How have the demographics of the neighborhood changed in the last five years?

☐ 1. More college students   (1)

☐ 2. More middle class residents   (2)

☐ 3. Fewer customers in general   (3)

☐ 4. None   (4)

D-2. Are you emotionally attached to your business?

☐ 1. Yes   (1)

☐ 2. No   (2)

D-3. Do you want to provide any additional information that may assist in this research?

Printed in the United States
By Bookmasters